ULCERS

M. Michael Eisenberg, M.D.

ULCERS

Random House **New York**

Copyright © 1978 by M. Michael Eisenberg, M.D.

All rights reserved under International and Pan-American Copyright Conventions.

Published in the United States by Random House, Inc., New York, and simultaneously in Canada by Random House of Canada Limited, Toronto.

Library of Congress Cataloging in Publication Data

Eisenberg, M. Michael, 1931–
Ulcers.

Bibliography: p.
Includes index.
1. Peptic ulcer.   I. Title.
RC821.E27   616.3'43   77–90315
ISBN 0–394–42753–X

Manufactured in the United States of America
2 4 6 8 9 7 5 3
First Edition

Acknowledgment is made to:

The Complete Poems of Emily Dickinson, edited by Thomas H. Johnson, 1960. On page 171.

Familiar Medical Quotations, edited by Maurice B. Strauss, 1st edition, 1968. Sir John Lubdock on page 119, E. C. MacDowell on page 209, Lawrence J. Henderson on page 82, Carl Jung on page 46, J. A. D. Anderson on page 46.

The University of Chicago Press: Excerpt From "How to Stay Young" by Leroy (Satchel) Paige quoted from *The Physiology and Treatment of Peptic Ulcer* by J. Garrott Allen, 611. © 1959 by The University of Chicago. Reprinted by permission.

IN MEMORY OF D.G.E.
—I KNOW SHE KNOWS

Acknowledgments

To my secretary, Gail Iverson, for her suggestions, patience and tireless retyping of the interminable revisions, I give my thanks.

And to CKE, EDE, EBE, and ACE for their long-suffering and sustained loyalty, I express wonderment and affection.

687 242

Foreword

The state of your health is determined as much by your individual makeup as by the external realities of your environment. Your susceptibility to peptic ulcer, perhaps more than any other health problem, is affected by your hormones, your personality, your reactions to stress, the food you eat, your life style, your family background, your politics and your philosophies. That some of us have ulcers is curious. The wonder is that we all don't.

On the most rudimentary level ulcers are caused when too much acid is produced by the stomach and the defenses of the gastrointestinal tract are too weak to handle it. But much more is involved in the ulcer process.

"No acid—no ulcer" is as true as anything we know about the disorder; but acid is only the last link in a long and unbelievably tangled chain of biological and social events that culminate in a final indignity—ulcer, a form of self-digestion by the stomach and its outlet, the duodenum.

In this book I'll explore many of the facets and nuances of the ailment. Impressions, conflicting interpretations, opinions, misconceptions, myths and legends abound, but I've tried to separate truth from fiction. Where existing information meets the strict requirements of the scientific process—where statistically significant population samples have been studied, where proven differences are apparent, where controls have been carefully structured, and where in my opinion interpretations of reported data have been intelligently analyzed—I've said so. When I feel these requirements haven't been met, you'll know that too.

By necessity I've made extensive use of statistics. They are marvelously flexible. You can do what you wish with them, and so can I. Statistics don't lie, they say, but statisticians do. I can show you that the average American has but one testicle and one female breast. I can tell you jokes about the statistician who drowned while wading across a stream of average depth of two feet. Or the one who carried a bomb on an airplane because the statistical likelihood of two people doing so was remote. Statistics can be weighted to convert yes to no and black to white. I'll do my best to judge them honestly, but my own bias is everywhere—in the studies I have chosen to quote, and in my analyses of what they mean. My between-the-lines insinuations and dogmatic views will color my judgment in ways that scientists aren't supposed to permit. There are simply too many "yes . . . but's" in the best of us, and I'm certainly not immune.

Readers may be inclined to ask such questions as "Does *he* have an ulcer? Is he a smoker? Does he drink alcohol? How about coffee? Does he have a family background of ulcers? Is his job stressful?" To put my own biases in somewhat better perspective, the answers to those questions are no, yes, rarely, no, no, and you better believe it.

This book is about much more than ulcers. It is about people, their behavior patterns and their responses. It's about the London blitz of World War II and about Norwegian fishermen. It's about Australian aspirin consumers and air traffic controllers at O'Hare Airport. It's about pregnant women and Little Leaguers. It tells of Abyssinian goatherds, New York taxi drivers and "executive" monkeys. I have woven the stories of people with ulcers throughout the entire fabric of the narrative. I learned the "facts" about ulcers in medical school, but I've learned about people with ulcers from people. You will too.

These are true stories and real people, many of whom I've known personally. I've borrowed some case studies from the writings of colleagues, and some are composites of several people. I have only changed names, places and a few inconsequential nonmedical details to protect their privacy. Any resemblance to people living or otherwise, however, *is* intended. You'll recognize them among your friends and family; their stories could be all our stories.

There are lessons to be learned, "tricks" to be tried, regimens that help and operations that cure. If you have an ulcer, think you have one, are afraid you're developing one or know someone who suffers from one, there is a chance—a likelihood, even—that pain and anxiety can be alleviated. At least, that's my intent.

People with ulcers have been an abiding concern of mine since the day I first thought I could understand why acid-pepsin causes ulcers. They've garnered my affection and they've evoked my enmity. They've rewarded me with the indescribable pleasure and ego enhancement of healing under my care, and they've frustrated me beyond description with their refusal to respond. I've attended their weddings, the christenings of their children, and on rare occasions, their wakes. I love them and they drive me to despair. But they are never boring. They have caught and held my attention. I believe they'll hold yours too.

xii

I dedicate this book, informally, to the thousands of clinical and laboratory investigators who have sought to unravel the truth, and to the people who have been the beneficiaries.

M.M.E.

Minneapolis and Taos
October 1977

Contents

4

taken are ten to fifteen aspirin a day for "stiffness in the joints." Now and then during the past week she has felt light-headed and dizzy, and she has noticed a peculiar and unfamiliar shiny black tarlike quality to her bowel movements. By evening her daughter, who checks on her daily, will have taken her to the emergency room at the university hospital, where the intern on call will admit her for diagnosis and treatment of profound anemia.

NEW YORK CITY. 10:50 A.M., THURSDAY, NOVEMBER 18, 1976

Since early this morning Cerise, a smashingly beautiful, well-groomed twenty-seven-year-old divorcee, a $60,000-a-year fashion photographer's model, has been posing under bright flood lamps. All she has eaten since last night are tea biscuits nibbled at increasingly frequent intervals. She hopes to suppress the growing mid-abdominal and back pain that has plagued her intermittently for almost a year. Her sex, social and professional life are all deteriorating. Within a few weeks her analyst will acknowledge that her symptoms are *not* due to a simple "nervous stomach" and will refer her to an internist for evaluation.

None of these people, of widely disparate ages and of different racial, genetic, social and economic backgrounds, bear much resemblance to the stereotype of a hard-driving, Gelusil-popping corporate executive. Yet they, along with an estimated ten or more million other Americans, all suffer from peptic ulcers.

To most laypeople the term "ulcers" conjures up a vision of belly pain brought on by stress and anxiety. To doctors, depending on their field of expertise, it can mean something quite different. To the ophthalmologist it may mean an abrasion of the cornea; to the dermatologist, a chronic or slowly healing break in the skin; and to the cardiologist, an eroded cholesterol plaque in a coronary artery or in a major leg vessel. To the gastroenterologist, who deals daily with the

Contents

xiv

CONTENTS

I

THE NATURE OF ULCERS

1

Ulcer Defined

ANAHEIM, CALIFORNIA. 7:26 P.M., TUESDAY, OCTOBER 26, 1976

Alton, a bright but somewhat intense black seventeen-year-old high school athlete and honor student, in peak physical condition, is studying for the Scholastic Aptitude Tests he is to take the next day. He's suddenly struck by an excruciating abdominal pain and collapses to the floor. His mother finds him, his face contorted in agony, lying in the fetal position. Within a few hours he'll be asleep on an operating table in a nearby hospital.

KANSAS CITY, KANSAS. 7:56 A.M., WEDNESDAY, OCTOBER 27, 1976

Emma, an eighty-eight-year-old Caucasian woman, a mild-mannered, rather sweet-natured former schoolteacher who's scarcely had a day's illness in her long life, is having trouble preparing her breakfast. The only medication she has ever taken are ten to fifteen aspirin a day for "stiffness in the joints." Now and then during the past week she has felt light-headed and dizzy, and she has noticed a peculiar and unfamiliar shiny black tarlike quality to her bowel movements. By evening her daughter, who checks on her daily, will have taken her to the emergency room at the university hospital, where the intern on call will admit her for diagnosis and treatment of profound anemia.

NEW YORK CITY. 10:50 A.M., THURSDAY, NOVEMBER 18, 1976

Since early this morning Cerise, a smashingly beautiful, well-groomed twenty-seven-year-old divorcee, a $60,000-a-year fashion photographer's model, has been posing under bright flood lamps. All she has eaten since last night are tea biscuits nibbled at increasingly frequent intervals. She hopes to suppress the growing mid-abdominal and back pain that has plagued her intermittently for almost a year. Her sex, social and professional life are all deteriorating. Within a few weeks her analyst will acknowledge that her symptoms are *not* due to a simple "nervous stomach" and will refer her to an internist for evaluation.

None of these people, of widely disparate ages and of different racial, genetic, social and economic backgrounds, bear much resemblance to the stereotype of a hard-driving, Gelusil-popping corporate executive. Yet they, along with an estimated ten or more million other Americans, all suffer from peptic ulcers.

To most laypeople the term "ulcers" conjures up a vision of belly pain brought on by stress and anxiety. To doctors, depending on their field of expertise, it can mean something quite different. To the ophthalmologist it may mean an abrasion of the cornea; to the dermatologist, a chronic or slowly healing break in the skin; and to the cardiologist, an eroded cholesterol plaque in a coronary artery or in a major leg vessel. To the gastroenterologist, who deals daily with the problems of the health and function of the gastrointestinal tract, it usually means peptic ulcer. And it's peptic ulcer with which we are going to concern ourselves.

Most people either know someone who has an ulcer or are afraid they may develop one themselves. Despite this, there is an enormous amount of misinformation and misunderstanding, as well as plain curiosity, about people with ulcers. There are also a great many questions about ulcers that people are reluctant to ask.

This is unfortunate, since the aggressive application of basic laboratory principles to patient care has reaped very impressive rewards in this area. Nearly a century of laboratory and clinical research has provided the medical profession with a much improved understanding of basic causes of ulcers and has helped to define groups of individuals especially at risk. Furthermore, this same information has contributed tremendously to the quality of treatment and consequently to the quality of life for those who suffer.

Peptic ulcer is a disorder of awesome social and economic impact. By midcentury in the United States the sales of prescription medications designed to suppress or neutralize acid production, and of over-the-counter preparations for "upset stomach," approximated 80 million dollars a year.*

Sir William Osler, the great diagnostician, characterized

---

* In the mid-fifties the combined loss of income due to total incapacitation by ulcer sufferers, the loss of their expected earnings as a result of premature death, and the expenses of medical care and hospitalization approached 500 million dollars annually. By the period from 1963 to 1965 the figure had risen to over a billion dollars. More importantly, the number of people developing a new ulcer each year rose 25 percent from the 1957–59 period to the 1963–65 one, and by that time over 3.5 million people yearly joined the ranks of ulcer sufferers. With the recent sharply inflated costs of medical care and the near doubling of per capita income, it's likely that these numbers are only modest estimates. The Stanford Research Institute estimates that in 1977 ulcer disease cost the nation 3.2 billion dollars, a 23 percent increase since 1975.

ulcer as the "wound stripe of Western civilization." It is not overstating the case to classify it as a major public health problem. More recent studies, however, show that the patterns of those who get ulcer and why are constantly changing.

Exact information on how many people presently suffer from ulcers and who they are is currently unavailable, partly because of poor record-keeping here and abroad in past times. Questionable accuracy in making the diagnosis further compounds the problem and makes a really precise analysis difficult. Still, there is solid evidence, from studies reported as far back as 1962, suggesting that by *that* time the yearly development of new ulcers in younger age groups had begun a decline; predictions were made that this decline would not only persist but would actually gain momentum.

This anticipated decrease in fact came true. In Great Britain by 1968 the annual rate of people developing new ulcers, in age groups from thirty-five to sixty-four, had fallen to half the levels observed only a decade before.

We don't have any ready explanations for these trends, and any pat interpretations are potentially erroneous. One theory has it that the influx of immigrants to America during the first half of this century increased the proportion of ulcer-prone people in the total population. The reasoning here is that these immigrants were a group of people under great stress and therefore particularly susceptible to ulcers. So as the great waves of immigration began to taper off after about three decades, the percentage of especially vulnerable people declined, although there were brief increases in postwar refugees in both 1945 and 1960. It follows that the downward trend in prevalence can be explained by a massive decrease in numbers of ulcer-prone people. While this theory may seem attractive at first, it's actually quite shaky. It doesn't explain why the same sort of decrease in the number of people with ulcers occurred in many other parts of the world as well as in the United States.

The decline was nevertheless real and can't be simply

pushed aside just because no neat explanation fits all the facts. But while the modern peak in incidence has passed, that's little consolation to the tens of millions who are currently suffering from the disorder or who will develop it in the coming years.

These observations are intriguing and tend to support what most of us already know intuitively. Peptic ulcer is a dynamic disorder—its incidence (the number of people who develop a new ulcer each year) and its prevalence (the number of people who already have ulcers) are related to a wide variety of social, economic, political and ecological factors. During periods of national or worldwide upheaval, a reversal in trend is both possible and likely.*

WHAT IS THE NATURE OF ULCERS?

From an anatomic viewpoint, an ulcer † is simply an open sore. It's not unlike a tiny crater or a minuscule volcano. It results from an inflammation and destruction of tissue in a very localized area. It's different from a wound made by a knife or by an abrasion, although this kind of injury can ulcerate too if it becomes infected.

A peptic ulcer is nonmalignant and is found in those portions of the gastrointestinal tract bathed by acid stomach juices. The usual peptic ulcer varies from a quarter to three-quarters of an inch in diameter, although much smaller and larger ones often occur.

For purposes of consistency, peptic ulcer will be defined as

---

* In fact a reversal may already have begun. In a report issued in February 1977, the Stanford Research Institute estimated that since 1968 ulcer prevalence has been increasing at the rate of 2.3 percent a year. The incidence rate per thousand population is also up.

† We commonly speak of people having *an* ulcer (singular) or ulcers (plural). Those terms will be used interchangeably, although in fact people usually have *an* ulcer rather than more than one.

an inflammatory sore in the lining of the gastrointestinal tract characterized by a loss of tissue, and by penetration at least through the entire lining and into the muscular coats of the stomach and intestine. Sometimes ulcers may completely penetrate the wall of the bowel, causing a through-and-through perforation.

Contrary to widespread belief, the stomach plays a relatively minor role in the digestive process. Its main functions are mechanical—food storage and the mixing of food with various gastric juices. The actual absorption of nutrients into the bloodstream is minimal in the stomach. At its lower end the stomach also regulates the process by which ingested food is delivered to the rest of the gastrointestinal tract. It's there, beyond the stomach, that the most important part of the digestive process—the absorption of food and its delivery to body tissues—takes place. Therefore, although an intact stomach is obviously desirable, the organ itself isn't essential to life.

One of the most important of the processes that go on in the stomach is the secretion of juices. In the development of peptic ulcer, the two key components of stomach juice are hydrochloric acid and the *pre*-enzyme pepsinogen. An enzyme is a substance secreted by the body's cells which acts as a catalyst to bring about certain chemical changes in other substances—for example, helping to decompose such organic materials as food.

Pepsinogen is inactive and harmless at alkaline or neutral levels. Under these conditions, it will not in any way cause digestion of food or damage of tissue. Hydrochloric acid is considerably more harmful than pepsinogen. Nevertheless, it will only damage animal tissue very slowly. Pepsinogen, when activated to the enzyme pepsin, becomes an extremely corrosive and damaging material capable of rapid digestion and destruction of the protein in practically all living tissue. This includes the walls of the stomach itself.

To convert pepsinogen to pepsin, the environment must

be very acid. Hydrochloric acid, secreted by the stomach and usually found in abundance in normal people, provides this environment. High acidity combined with very small amounts of pepsin makes pure gastric juice one of the most injurious and caustic of the body's secretions.

For years after the digestive and corrosive character of the gastric juice was recognized and the roles of acid and pepsin understood, considerable controversy surrounded the relative importance of each. However, any distinction between the two is both artificial and misleading. Since the substances are interdependent for their digestive action, the question of which is dominant is really irrelevant. It is cliché in medical circles to quote the rule of thumb "No acid, no ulcer." It would be just as appropriate to claim "No *pepsin,* no ulcer—either!"

Under normal conditions the membrane lining the gastrointestinal tract is well shielded from the virulent effects of activated gastric juice. A host of defensive mechanisms keep the stomach from digesting itself or any other part of the intestines with which these secretions may come in contact. In fact, it's a tribute to this protective apparatus that we don't all have peptic ulcer.

Sometimes, however, these normally present protective barriers break down. Sometimes they are inadequate to begin with. Other times they are simply overwhelmed by the digestive juices. One theory concerning the cause of peptic ulcer suggests that large amounts of acid in the stomach may first attack some of the protective mechanisms. This then exposes the mucous lining of the stomach or small intestine to pepsin, resulting in peptic ulcer.

Most people with peptic ulcer make too much acid for their defenses to handle. Peptic ulcer results from an imbalance between the secretion of damaging digestive juices on the one hand and the capacity of the protective processes to defend against these secretions, on the other. The consequence is gastrointestinal self-destruction and auto-digestion.

It's easy to see why all modern treatment for ulcer, whether applied by the internist or the surgeon, is directed at suppression or neutralization of the acid stomach juices.

Peptic ulcer is a general term applicable to *any* ulcer resulting from the contact of body tissues with active gastric juice. The ulcer may even occur on the skin when a puncture (fistula) occurs between the stomach and the surface of the body. This can result, for example, from a gunshot wound. Certainly no part of the gastrointestinal tract is immune from the devastating effects of acid-pepsin. Peptic ulcers can be found in the esophagus, stomach, duodenum and small bowel, and under unusual circumstances, even the large bowel (colon). However, our discussions concerning ulcers will be directed at the two most common sites: (1) the stomach itself (gastric ulcer), and (2) the first portion of the small intestine leading away from the stomach—the duodenum (duodenal ulcer).

DUODENAL ULCER

Most people think the most common site of peptic ulcer is the stomach. Many sufferers say, "I have stomach ulcers." This is a misconception. Duodenal ulcer is five to ten times more common than gastric ulcer, and is usually found in the duodenal bulb. (See the figure on page 25.) Why this particular area should have such a strong predilection for ulcer is not entirely clear.

Duodenal ulcer is a disorder primarily of adulthood, though we are finding it more and more frequently in children. No age is free from the disease; the youngest ulcer patient I have seen is a three-month-old infant, and the oldest, a ninety-three-year-old man. It has been reported in the newborn and even in the unborn child still in its mother's womb.

Ulcers are far more common in men than in women: depending on the area of the world and the population sample being studied, duodenal ulcers can occur up to ten times as often in males. Duodenal ulcer is a lifetime disorder. Although there may be long periods of remission, during which time the ulcer becomes dormant and symptoms completely disappear, these respites are usually temporary. Sooner or later, unless medical therapy is intensive and continuous or unless the acid overproduction is permanently controlled by surgery, the ulcer tends to flare up again and again. I have encountered hundreds of people with ten, twenty, thirty or even more years of intermittent ulcer activity.

Duodenal ulcer most commonly develops between ages sixteen and twenty-five, although from adolescence on, it's a common disorder.

Jason is a fairly typical example.

CHICAGO, ILLINOIS. MARCH 12, 1974

Jason, a thirty-seven-year-old Caucasian male, is an ambitious and hard-working $65,000-a-year attorney. He has been happily married for about nine and a half years, and has two small children. His special interest is corporate tax law, and he is very good at it. His hobbies include tennis, golf, skiing, and photography. He is quite congenial, polite, and rather more easy to get along with than one might expect from such an intense person. No one has ever seen him lose his temper at the office, and he invariably presents a calm and courteous exterior to the public. He is regarded by both his colleagues and the people who work for him as something of a perfectionist, and the standards he sets for himself and for others are very high.

He no longer smokes; he drinks alcohol only occasionally. He has no more than five or six cups of decaffeinated coffee a day, and the only medicine he takes on a regular basis is an acid-neutralizing substance.

He was in excellent health until his second year of college. During his college years he studied diligently, smoking up to two packs of cigarettes a day; he averaged ten to fifteen cups of coffee daily; he often skipped meals and virtually never had breakfast. He noticed a gradually increasing number of "hunger pains" during his sophomore year. These were easily and quickly relieved by food or milk. But by the time he entered Columbia Law School his "hunger pains" were so frequent and intense that he finally sought medical advice.

Physical examination was normal. So were his blood tests. His blood type was determined to be O positive. His body build was lean and muscular. His family history was generally unremarkable except for the fact that his father and an uncle both suffered from ulcers.

Based on the history of his complaints, his physician, a thorough and experienced practitioner, ordered an upper gastrointestinal barium x-ray study, a telescopic examination of his stomach and duodenum (endoscopy), and measurements of the rate at which his stomach makes acid. The x-rays showed distortion of his duodenal bulb with a small active ulcer crater in the center of scar tissue. Endoscopic examination confirmed the presence of the ulcer in the scar. Acid secretion was measured at two and a half times normal for his age and sex.

He was placed on acid-neutralizing and -suppressing medication. A bland diet was also prescribed. He was ordered to cut down on his smoking, to eliminate alcohol temporarily from his daily routine, to minimize caffeine intake, and to avoid aspirin and aspirin-containing medication, including the so-called buffered compounds.

He's done moderately well since that time. He loses only two or three days a year due to pain and discomfort. In general, his ulcer has remained under relatively satisfactory control; he has learned to live with it. But when he deviates from the prescribed therapy program, if only for a week or two, it costs him dearly. His ulcer flares up to its previous intensity.

The life history of this very pleasant and accomplished man incorporates many of the features supposedly typical of people with duodenal ulcer. He is a lean, muscular

Caucasian male. He is future-oriented and conscientious. His ulcer first developed when he was young. Both his father and uncle had ulcers. His blood group is type O; he makes two and a half times the normal amount of stomach acid; and while his ulcer can be controlled with therapy, it flares up and subsides irregularly but unremittently.

GASTRIC ULCER

The second most common form of peptic ulcer is gastric ulcer. Like duodenal ulcer, it is caused by self-digestion, but it has several features that differentiate it from duodenal ulcer. Gastric ulcer is always found in the stomach itself— usually, but not always, on the right side or lesser curvature of the stomach—while duodenal ulcer is most often found at or just beyond the junction of the stomach and duodenum.

Gastric ulcer is only about one-fourth as common as duodenal ulcer, but in a high percentage of cases (up to 40 percent) it is found *in conjunction with* duodenal ulcer. This is called "combined" or "double" ulcer. Like duodenal ulcer, it is sometimes, though relatively less often, seen in children. However, unlike duodenal ulcer, not only is gastric ulcer primarily an adult disease, but it develops when people are in their forties, fifties, sixties, or even older.

Gastric and duodenal ulcers are both predominantly male diseases. But duodenal ulcer is five to ten times more common in men than in women, while gastric ulcer is only two or three times more common. The dictum "No acid, no ulcer" does hold for both types, but the levels of acid secretion in the person with gastric ulcer are lower, tending to be normal or even subnormal.

The complications of gastric ulcer, such as bleeding or perforation, are less well tolerated than those of duodenal ulcer, partly because gastric ulcer tends to occur in older people. Because the kinds of surgery that work well for people with duodenal ulcer don't work as well with gastric-ulcer patients, doctors use a different operation to meet their special requirements.

George is a typical gastric-ulcer candidate.

MINNEAPOLIS, MINNESOTA. FEBRUARY 23, 1977

George is a sixty-two-year-old Caucasian male. He works on an auto assembly line at the local Ford plant, earning $18,000 a year with overtime. A reliable and conscientious worker, he has missed work only four days in twenty years. By nature he is easygoing, pleasant, mild-mannered and generous. Unfortunately, only three months earlier, his wife of forty years died after a long siege with cancer. George was a devoted family man, but with his three sons grown and married and his wife now gone, he is desperately lonely. He was an avid hunter, fisherman and amateur restorer of antique cars. However, he is having a hard time adjusting to his new existence. He has lost interest in eating and has lost seventeen pounds in thirteen weeks.

He smokes two or three twenty-cent cigars a day. A six-pack of beer lasts him a week. He drinks five or six cups of coffee a day, always with meals. He takes no medications of any kind.

George has always enjoyed excellent health and has always regarded himself as robust. Though he has always had specific food preferences, almost nothing ever upset his stomach. But he hasn't been feeling at all well for almost two months. Abdominal pain has plagued him frequently since a month after his wife's death. Food and drink don't bring lasting relief—as a matter of fact, they sometimes make his pain worse. He's tried various over-the-counter antacids, all with indifferent results. It's time to seek medical advice.

Physical examination is essentially normal. His blood pressure is slightly elevated. Blood tests show a moderate anemia, with a hemoglobin of 9.5 grams (normal is 12.5–14.0 grams). An examination of his stool reveals evidence of microscopic amounts of blood. His blood group type is A negative.

The family history is basically unrevealing except for the fact that his brother, now dead, was thought to have had a stomach ulcer.

Based on the history of complaints, the weight loss, the anemia and the finding of blood in the stool, admission to the hospital for careful evaluation was advised. A battery of tests were carried out, including: an x-ray of the upper gastrointestinal tract; a barium enema of the colon; endoscopy of the esophagus, stomach and duodenum, with biopsy; measurements of his stomach's rate of acid secretion; and a search of the stomach juices for malignant cells.

The x-rays showed a nonmalignant-appearing ulcer of the lesser curve of the stomach; endoscopy confirmed the diagnosis of gastric ulcer and all biopsies were negative for cancer. Studies of his acid secretion revealed a rate of production only half normal for his age and his sex. Microscopic examination of the stomach juices revealed no malignant cells.

George will be placed on a bland diet. He is to avoid all alcoholic and caffeine-containing beverages. He may continue smoking one or two cigars a day. He will be given a mood elevator, and acid-neutralizing medication to be taken on an intensive fourteen-hour-a-day schedule. He will be encouraged to take a short vacation—to go hunting and fishing with his oldest grandson. In six weeks he will be examined again and will undergo the same tests.

If by that time the ulcer has healed by 50 percent or more, he will be given an additional "test of healing" for another four weeks. If it has not, he will be offered surgery. The chances that he will be operated on some time during the next five years approaches 80 percent. Even if his ulcer heals during the initial trial, it is almost certain to recur.

George is a fairly typical example of a person with benign gastric ulcer, although there are many variations to the syndrome. He is elderly, male and Caucasian, belongs to blood group type A, and has recently been under stress. He makes less than the normal amount of acid for someone of his age and sex; his brother may have had gastric ulcer; his ulcer came late in life; relief by antacids and food is incomplete, and sometimes meals aggravate the discomfort. George will probably eventually require surgery for permanent control of the ulcer.

You can see that there are fundamental differences between ulcers of the duodenum and those which occur in the stomach. In fact, these two types of peptic ulcer seem to represent different diseases. The chart below shows the distinct characteristics of each.

DUODENAL ULCER	GASTRIC ULCER
1. Occurs in younger people.	Tends to occur in older people.
2. Is predominantly associated with greater than normal amounts of acid.	Is usually associated with normal or less than normal amounts of acid.
3. Occurs in higher social and economic classes.	Occurs in lower social and economic classes.
4. Has a high association with blood group type O.	Has a higher than normal association with blood group type A.
5. Is associated with intellectually demanding jobs and high-anxiety personalities.	Is associated with jobs that require heavy physical activity, often under unusual climatic, environmental and geographic circumstances.
6. Eating often relieves symptoms.	Food frequently causes discomfort.
7. The stomach is often hyperactive and has a greater than normal number of acid-secreting cells.	The stomach is often sluggish and has fewer than normal acid-producing cells.
8. Is a predominantly male disorder.	Ratio of male to female sufferers is relatively low.

DUODENAL ULCER	GASTRIC ULCER
9. Responds well to operations in which the vagus nerves are cut (see chapters 2 and 14).	Responds better to operations in which part of the stomach, including the ulcer, is removed.

It will be helpful to keep these distinctions in mind as we examine the possible causes of ulcers, in the chapters to come.

PEPTIC ULCER AND CANCER

One would think that the pain and discomfort caused by peptic ulcer would be burden enough for people to bear, but fear and anxiety concerning the possibility that ulcer is in fact cancer or may lead to cancer is frequently an overriding concern. Even after I have explained peptic ulcer in detail to patients and their families, I often get the response: "Yes, Doctor—we understand. But tell me the truth, it isn't cancer, is it?" Therefore it seems to me that the relationship between nonmalignant peptic ulcer and cancerous ulcer should be commented upon.

There's absolutely no evidence that peptic duodenal ulcer causes cancer. Cancer of the duodenum is extremely uncommon, and even though the precise causes for its development aren't clear, no link has ever been established with duodenal ulcer. People who have been suffering from duodenal ulcer for thirty or even more years probably do not have an increased risk of developing malignancy in this area.

On the other hand, as far as peptic *gastric* ulcer is concerned, the situation is a little harder to assess. Controversy has surrounded the possible cause-and-effect relationship between long-standing gastric ulcer and cancer for nearly a century. In the medical literature, the reported incidence of cancerous breakdown of a gastric ulcer has varied from *never* to *always*. There are studies stating that anywhere from 5 to

15 percent of gastric ulcers are associated with malignancy, but clinical experience throughout the world doesn't confirm this.

An important distinction has to be made between benign gastric ulcers that become cancerous and cancers that are already present. Some stomach cancers can be partially digested by gastric juices in much the same way as the normal stomach lining can. These may resemble ordinary peptic ulcer. But it doesn't mean that the cancer developed from the ulcer. Quite the contrary—it may well be that the malignant tissue, because of its poor quality and its relatively scanty blood supply and nutrition, is more easily digested by gastric juices. Examiners may mistakenly think that the tumor is growing at the edge of a benign ulcer when what they are actually seeing is a cancer being slowly digested by stomach enzymes. Even in the absence of acid, a cancer may break down or disintegrate to form an ulcer. This is not a peptic ulcer; it's a malignant one.

The fact that this controversy exists, however, should raise a red flag for both the person with stomach ulcers and the physician. About 4 percent of stomach ulcers are already malignant. It must therefore be determined promptly whether *any* gastric ulcer is or is not already a cancer. For this reason the proper diagnostic evaluation of a patient with gastric ulcer must include endoscopic examination of his or her stomach, with biopsies of the ulcer. Stomach acid secretion studies performed at the same time can also help. Except under very rare circumstances, the person with benign gastric ulcer always makes some acid. About six out of every ten patients with gastric cancer, however, can't make acid. If the patient has an ulcer and his stomach is shown to be incapable of making acid, the diagnosis of cancer must be seriously considered. More aggressive testing, such as a search for loose cancer cells in the stomach juices, can be carried out. Kristjan's case illustrates these points.

HOUSTON, TEXAS. JANUARY 14, 1970

Kristjan is a forty-three-year-old blond (almost white-haired), blue-eyed male physician born and raised in rugged terrain sixty miles from Reykjavík, Iceland. For the past year he has been on sabbatical at the University of Texas Medical School. Six days ago Kristjan noticed mild abdominal pain in his upper mid-abdomen; this pain has persisted. Kristjan is genuinely alarmed, for Icelandic males have the highest rate of stomach cancer in the world. This is possibly related to the remarkably homogeneous population, or perhaps to the country's diet, which is very heavy in smoked fish.

He promptly seeks the aid of a fellow physician, who examines him and orders gastrointestinal x-ray studies and some blood tests. The stomach film shows a small irregular crater located high on the greater curvature of the stomach, an unusual site for benign gastric ulcer. Endoscopy is performed the same day, and the lesion, which appears to the examiner as indeterminate insofar as benignity or malignancy is concerned, is biopsied. Acid secretion studies are made, and washings of the stomach taken for microscopic examination.

Kristjan's worst fears are confirmed. His stomach makes normal amounts of acid, but both the washings and the biopsies show malignant cells. He is promptly admitted to the hospital, is prepared for surgery, and within seventy-two hours undergoes an operation for removal of his stomach.

There is no evidence of tumor spread; the lesion is small and shows malignancy only at the edges. He stands about a one-in-two chance of being free of recurrence over the next five years.

Kristjan's story, though not yet complete, is nevertheless encouraging. Prompt medical attention, an accurate diagnosis and skillful treatment, combined with the early nature of his malignancy, have given him the best chance for long-term survival. He remains well and free of cancer recurrence more than seven years later.

If your physician tells you that you have a gastric ulcer, you should be reassured by every diagnostic measure available that it is not a cancer. Even if you undergo ulcer surgery a diligent search for microscopic evidence of tumor must be made. This is a routine precaution.

2

How Your Stomach and Duodenum Work

Some have made the stomach a mill; some would have it to be a stewing pot; and some a wort-trough; yet all the while one would have thought that it must have been very evident, that the stomach was neither a mill, nor a stewing pot, nor a wort-trough, nor anything but a stomach.
—William Hunter (1718–1783)

When most of us complain of a "stomach ache," we usually mean that we have a pain in our abdomen. However, the abdomen is an area housing many organs, any of which can be the source of the discomfort. Even doctors, nurses and medical students commonly use the words "abdomen," "belly" and "stomach" interchangeably, so ingrained are the habits of everyday speech. Take the following example:

LONG ISLAND CITY, NEW YORK. AUGUST 25, 1975

Cynthia is a thirty-three-year-old Caucasian housewife. She's the mother of five children under the age of twelve. Slightly obese, she has nevertheless been basically well all of her life. But for the past two weeks she's been complaining of a pain on the right side under her ribs, especially after eating. Twice in the last five nights she's been awakened by her discomfort.

Managing the somewhat chaotic household and her other obligations have kept her from seeking medical advice. Like most of us, she tends to deny—even to herself—that anything serious is going on, and hope triumphs over reality. She believes that if she ignores her pain long enough it will disappear.

However, because her symptoms persist and her husband and friends insist, she finally presents herself to the family physician, telling him that she "has a stomach ache."

In fact, Cynthia's pain isn't arising from her stomach at all. She's suffering from a chronic inflammation of the gallbladder. She has gallstones. Detailed physical examination, laboratory studies and x-rays by her physician will eliminate most of the common causes of abdominal pain; the gallbladder will be incriminated as the most likely cause of her symptoms, and she'll be treated accordingly.

Because Cynthia is young and basically healthy and since we don't at present have a sound method for dissolving gallstones, she'll be advised to have surgery. Her gallbladder will be removed together with the stones, and she'll be completely and permanently relieved of her problems.

The abdomen is really nothing more than a space bounded at the top by the diaphragm (which separates it from the organs of the chest—the heart and lungs and the great vessels), and at the bottom by the inlet to the pelvis and the pelvic organs. It is bounded at the front by the muscles of the abdominal wall, and at the rear by the back of the ribs, the spinal column and the muscular walls of the flanks. Within the abdominal cavity are the liver, gallbladder, a short segment of the esophagus, the stomach, the small and large bowel, the pancreas and the spleen. The kidneys lie behind the abdominal space, fixed to the back wall.

The pelvic organs, which are also a potential source of bellyache, consist of the uterus, Fallopian tubes, ovaries, bladder and lower portion of the large bowel in the female; the bladder, the prostate and the lower part of the large bowel in the male.

In our discussions concerning people with ulcer, almost all our attention will be directed at the organs in which the disorder is most commonly found—the esophagus, the stomach, and the outlet from the stomach, the duodenum. Fortunately the form and the function of these three organs is relatively simple and easy to understand. Figures 1 and 2 will help you familiarize yourself with their general shape and some of their basic functions. Figure 1 is labeled from an anatomical (form) point of view, while Figure 2 describes the physiology (function) of the various areas.

THE ESOPHAGUS

The esophagus, or gullet, is a muscular tube about one inch in diameter and approximately ten to twelve inches in length. It passes from the mouth and back of the throat (pharynx) through the back part of the neck, chest and upper abdomen to the stomach. It acts as a channel for swallowed solids, liquids and air. These materials are propelled downward by a very effective series of sequential and orderly muscular contractions (peristalsis).

The inner lining of the esophageal wall is a rather delicate membrane called the mucosa, similar to that which lines the entire gastrointestinal tract from mouth to anus. The esophageal mucosa differs from the mucosa in other areas mainly in the cells, which secrete only a small amount of thin watery mucus. The juices of the esophagus play essentially no role in the digestive process.

The entire length of the mucosa is surrounded by a loose connective tissue called the submucosa, through which course many of the small vessels that bring nutrients to the inner lining and lend it support. The outer two layers of the esophageal tube consist of an inner circular muscle, which completely surrounds the mucosa and submucosa, and an outer longitudinal muscle, both of which extend from the back of the throat to the end of the esophagus, where they blend with the muscular coats of the stomach.

Particularly at its lower end, the esophageal lining is subject to peptic ulceration, just as is any other mucosal surface of the gastrointestinal tract that comes in contact with activated stomach juices. However, ulcers here are far less common than ulcers in the stomach and duodenum, because the small amount of acid gastric juice normally regurgitated during eating or changes in position (when you bend over, for example) is quickly cleared by a swallow or two of saliva.

The lower end of the esophagus where it joins with the stomach acts like a one-way valve. This gate mechanism is quite ingenious; the passage of foods and liquids into the stomach is normally unimpeded, but the valve won't permit the stomach contents back up into the esophagus.

Some medical conditions, such as hiatus hernia, involve a faulty valve that permits a two-way flow of material. This can cause inflammation and peptic ulceration of the esophagus.

THE STOMACH

The stomach varies considerably in size and shape from person to person and from time to time within the same person. It is a muscular sac capable of comfortably holding approxi-

Upper Gastrointestinal
ANATOMY

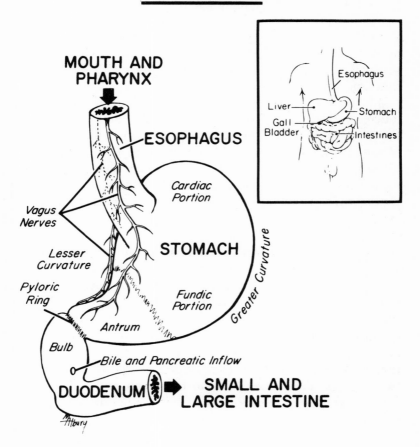

mately one quart of fluid or food. But it can undergo tremendous dilation and expansion, and under certain circumstances it can accommodate a much larger volume.

Cardiac Portion: The upper portion of the stomach, at the point where the esophagus joins it, is called the cardia. The stomach is relatively thin-walled in this area. The cardia functions largely as a storage bin.

The cardia is lined with a mucosa that primarily secretes mucus, a thin, somewhat slimy material that helps protect the stomach mucosa. The cells carpeting the cardiac portion of the mucosa are also capable of secreting acid and pepsin. Since the combination of acid and pepsin destroys unprotected gastrointestinal lining, the mucus acts as a kind of watershed, separating free acid and pepsin from direct contact with the cells.

The Fundus: The cardiac portion of the stomach runs into the fundus portion; the actual junction between the two areas is indistinct and arbitrary. The fundic portion of the stomach is the most spacious, allows for the greatest distension, and provides the most storage area. It, too, is lined with a mucosa capable of secreting acid and pepsin. Mucus is also produced here, but to a lesser extent than in the cardiac portion. Muscular activity in this portion of the stomach mixes the food and fluid received from the esophagus with gastric juices, and passes them on into the duodenum and lower intestines.

The Antrum: This is the lowest portion of the stomach, making up approximately a quarter of the entire organ. In many ways, the antrum is the most complex part of the stomach. It's the most heavily muscled section. As such, it acts as a pump, not only helping churn and mix food, liquid and gastric juices but also pushing the mixed food and liquids through the valve at the lower end of the stomach.

The cells making up the antral mucosal lining have a highly specialized function: the manufacture and secretion of the hormone gastrin, a key stimulus to the production of both gastric acid and pepsin. No acid or pepsin is produced in the antrum. Mucus is manufactured there, but this is a relatively minor function.

The Pylorus: The part of the stomach farthest from the mouth, the outlet called the pylorus, is a muscular fibrous ring that acts as a one-way valve in regulating the emptying of the stomach. The term "pylorus" is in fact derived from the Greek word meaning "gate-keeper."

Blood Vessels: The blood supply to the esophagus, stomach and duodenum is of course important, but from the point of view of people with ulcers the detailed anatomy of the vessels in these areas is of no particular interest in terms of the ulcer process except for the fact that these organs are richly supplied. Ulcers penetrating deeply enough into the walls of these organs may digest a hole in a large vessel and give rise to significant bleeding.

The single most important artery in this regard is called the gastro-duodenal vessel; it passes behind the duodenum precisely in the area where duodenal ulcer is most commonly found. Erosion into this vessel can cause frightening hemorrhage.

Nerves: The nerves supplying the stomach are of particular interest. They play a major role not only in the muscular or motor function of the stomach but also in the production of acid and peptic juices. They are therefore a key to the control of secretion of these juices. The most important of these, the vagus nerves, stem from the brain itself, passing out of the skull downward and branching out to supply the pharynx, esophagus, stomach, duodenum and upper and

Upper Gastrointestinal
FUNCTION

ORAL INTAKE

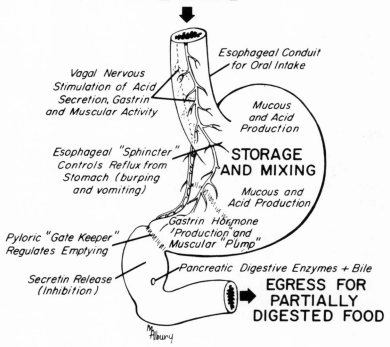

Esophageal Conduit
for Oral Intake

Vagal Nervous
Stimulation of Acid
Secretion, Gastrin
and Muscular Activity

Mucous
and Acid
Production

Esophageal "Sphincter"
Controls Reflux from
Stomach (burping
and vomiting)

STORAGE
AND MIXING

Mucous and
Acid Production

Gastrin Hormone
Production and
Muscular "Pump"

Pyloric "Gate Keeper"
Regulates Emptying

Pancreatic Digestive Enzymes + Bile

Secretin Release
(Inhibition)

EGRESS FOR
PARTIALLY
DIGESTED FOOD

M.
Albury

lower intestines, as well as the liver, pancreas and gall-bladder.

THREE CLASSICAL PHASES OF STOMACH FUNCTION

Since the turn of the century, when the famous Russian physiologist Ivan Pavlov did his most important work on dogs, stomach function has been described as occurring in three separate phases.

Cephalic Phase: The first of these, the cephalic or "brain" phase, depends on our conscious recognition of the sight, smell or taste of food. The brain then sends messages by way of the vagus nerves to other organs below. The mouth waters and the stomach prepares to receive swallowed material.

Gastric Phase: This next phase is characterized by the release of the hormone gastrin from the antrum portion of the stomach. Acid and pepsin start to flow and the stomach churns and mixes its contents into a "chyme" or blend of juices, food, saliva and mucus, readying it to be passed on to the lower intestines. Very little absorption of food takes place in the stomach, but water and some drugs such as alcohol *can* be absorbed.

Intestinal Phase: Finally, after food, liquid and acid-pepsin pass through the pylorus, various hormones are released from the duodenum and upper intestine to inhibit the activity going on above.

A Cybernetic Mechanism: Even though it's convenient to think of the stomach's function as occurring in three separate phases, all of the phases occur simultaneously and are interrelated in complex ways. Inhibiting and stimulating factors combine to make up an effective and smooth-working cybernetic mechanism. The brain sees, smells and tastes food and sends impulses down the vagus nerves to the stomach. The stomach starts to churn and releases gastrin, which, along with the nerve impulses, causes acid to flow. The gastrin also closes the valve between the esophagus and stomach so that the churning doesn't force gastric contents to back up. The pyloric gate-keeper at the lower end of the stomach relaxes, and the mixed contents pass on to the duodenum. If the stomach makes too much acid or passes the material on through too fast, gastrin and acid production slow down, the muscular churning decreases, hormones from the duodenum tighten the gate-keeper, and the whole process begins again in an orderly fashion.

The vagus nerves and the hormone gastrin are the two most important stimuli to the secretion of acid by the stomach. Not only do they individually have a direct effect on acid production, but they also sensitize the acid-secreting apparatus to each other and to other stimuli as well.

The essence of controlling acid—and therefore ulcers—is the restraint of these two stimuli. All modern medical and surgical treatment of ulcers is directed toward this end.

II

THE
ULCER-PRONE
PERSON

3

The Ulcer Susceptibility Test

Some elements in our makeup can be clearly identified as causing ulcers. Making too much stomach acid is one. Taking large amounts of aspirin is another. A third is our genetic legacy. Some of these forces are within our grasp to modify and control, while others obviously are not. Some of the other elements that go into the make-up of the ulcer-prone person are less clearly defined, such as the role your personality plays, the kind of work you do, how you play, what you eat and where you live, just to mention a few. While each element may individually exert only a small influence on who gets ulcers and why, when taken together in pairs or groups, they seem to contribute more convincingly to a setting in which ulcers develop, like weeds in an otherwise orderly garden.

Our goal will be to examine as many of the known po-

THE ULCER SUSCEPTIBILITY TEST

Factors That Appear to Affect the Vulnerability of People to Ulcers

+/– of questionable importance
+ possibly important
++ likely important
+++ clearly important

	Factors	Type	Score	Things which seem to help
1.	Male: Between the ages of sixteen and twenty-five	Duodenal	+++	See chapters 11 through 16.
	Male: Age forty and over	Gastric	+++	
2.	Female: Between the ages of sixteen and thirty and in life-crisis situations	Duodenal Gastric	++ +/–	Pregnancy helps. Diet, mood, self-esteem and quitting job, of possible value only. See chapters 9 and 11–16.
	Female: After menopause (whether natural or induced by surgery)	Duodenal (flare-up) Gastric (new)	++ ++	
3.	High levels of acid and pepsin in stomach juices	Duodenal Gastric	+++ +/–	Suppression of acid by medication or surgery. See chapters 14, 15 and 16.
4.	Family history of a close relative with ulcer	Duodenal Gastric	+++ +++	See Chapter 8.
5.	Blood group type O Blood group type A	Duodenal Gastric	++ +	See Chapter 7.
6.	Race: Caucasian Negroid Oriental	Duodenal or Gastric	+/– +/– +/–	See Chapter 7.
7.	Personality characteristics	Duodenal	++	See Chapter 5 and Afterword.
8.	Heavy intake of aspirin	Gastric Duodenal	+++ +	Aspirin avoidance or substitutes.
	Heavy intake of alcohol, tobacco, coffee, cola	Duodenal Gastric	+/– +/–	Moderation? See Chapter 6.
9.	High socioeconomic status Low socioeconomic status	Duodenal Gastric	+ +	See chapters 4, 7.

THE ULCER SUSCEPTIBILITY TEST

	Factors	Type	Score	Things which seem to help
10.	Children with stressful home environments, parental discord	Duodenal	++	Stabilized environment? See Chapter 10.
11.	Suppressed anger and high anxiety. Personal interpretation of the environment as stressful.	Duodenal	++	Anger-out? See Chapter 5.
		Gastric	+/−	
12.	Stressfully interpreted occupations	Duodenal	+	Job change? See Chapter 4.
		Gastric	+	
13.	Dietary factors	Duodenal	+	Avoidance of foods that cause discomfort. Strict diet during flare-up. See Chapter 13.
		Gastric	+	
14.	Rejection, expulsion or voluntary exclusion from a group or institution	Duodenal	+	See chapters 5, 7.
		Gastric	+/−	
15.	Geography, altitude, season, time of month, week, day. War, political unrest, economic crises	Duodenal	+	See Chapter 7.
		Gastric	+	

tentiators of ulcers as possible, to consider them separately and together, and to weigh their importance in making some people more, or less, vulnerable to ulcers. Above is a chart of the features commonly considered significant when one is trying to define the ulcer-prone "type."

You'll notice that I have assigned a relative weight to these fifteen factors, in terms of what we know of their individual significance. Be careful not to take these quantitations too literally. In any given individual they may have more or less influence than I have suggested, depending on what *other* elements are present. For example, lots of people have a family history of ulcers but never develop one themselves. But if a person with a family history of ulcers is male and belongs to blood group type O, his chances of getting an ulcer are increased. If he also makes too much acid, the risk rises still higher. And if he takes large amounts of aspirin on a regular basis, the potential for the development of an ulcer soars, and possibility becomes probability or even likelihood.

Using this profile as a guide, we will examine in finer detail the fifteen elements that contribute to having ulcers in order to gain a fuller understanding of the ulcer-prone person and to discover some ways in which the patterns can be modified and the risks lowered.

4

Your Job as a Cause of Ulcer

The mass of men lead lives of quiet desperation.
—Henry David Thoreau, *Walden*

Almost everyone associates certain kinds of jobs with ulcers. Some refer to the disorder as the "Wall Street disease." Others see Madison Avenue as a pressure cooker for ulcers. Most executives think of themselves as especially vulnerable, and "this job is giving me ulcers" is almost universal in their jargon.

Stop any ten people and ask them to describe those who are likely to suffer from ulcers; a remarkably consistent popular image emerges. Over and over again you'll hear adjectives like ambitious, hard-driving, intense, anxious, perfectionist, responsible, harried, worried, twitchy, demanding, self-critical and exacting. Ask about the kinds of jobs these people hold, and you will be told that they are advertising execu-tives, presidents of major businesses, frenetic press agents, overworked attorneys, military officers, high-powered sur-geons, politicians, prosperous salesmen and "leaders."

The conventional notion is that the ulcer-prone person is a successful, tyrannical perfectionistic workaholic. In short, you'll be told that these are the people who make the deci-sions in our society.

J. J. Groen, a psychiatrist, has stated that the fast pace of our contemporary civilization has imposed burdens on us that don't exist in most other cultures. Nor did they exist in Western culture prior to industrialization. In bygone eras, and even today in some less Westernized cultures, the rung of the social ladder on which you are born is the one on which you remain, no matter how hard you may try to climb to the top. In our culture today, however, upward mobility is a realistic goal.

M. Pflanz, a German scientist who's written extensively on the social aspects of ulcer, has pointed out that many epi-demiologic studies of psychosomatic disorders (of which duo-denal ulcer is probably the most common) are made up of loose generalizations based on a few intensively studied cases that aren't very convincing; often the group of people being studied isn't matched with a control group composed of those who do not suffer from the ailment. In reaching their conclusions researchers often fail to take into consideration social, economic, nutritional, racial, sexual, age, climatic and other influences that may be at play.

These shaky generalizations sometimes gain widespread acceptance. For example, a now classic study on the develop-ment of duodenal ulcers in monkeys was reported in 1958 by R. W. Porter and his associates at the Division of Neuropsy-chiatry, Walter Reed Army Institute of Research. These sci-entists noted an unusually high incidence of gastrointestinal disease in a group of monkeys undergoing experiments designed to analyze certain features of emotional behavior. In one part of the investigation, two pairs of monkeys matched for size, weight and sex were strapped into chairs. After a pair was exposed to a flashing red light, a painful electric shock was administered to their feet. One animal in each pair (the experimental or decision-making monkey) could prevent the shock for both itself and its partner (the control or passive monkey) by pressing on a bar.

After considerable training the experimental monkey learned to do this. If she failed to press the bar in time, both she and her partner were shocked. The number of shocks administered and the time intervals involved were the same for all the animals. Since the control monkey's lever was ineffective, she exerted no influence over her environment. For the most part she lost interest in her dummy lever. The death of the *experimental* monkey ended the study in both cases; one died from a perforated and the other from a penetrating duodenal ulcer.

The authors were careful not to overinterpret these observations. No firm conclusions could be drawn concerning the relationship between anxiety, mental fatigue and the development of ulcer. The researchers realized that loss of sleep and actual physical deterioration resulting from the intense experimental procedure could have caused the ulcers in the decision-making monkeys, rather than the "anxiety stress" of decision-making.

Descriptions of this fascinating experiment are available in dozens of textbooks and in many articles devoted to the subject of stress as a cause of duodenal ulcers. In all these discussions the experimental monkey is invariably referred to as the "executive" monkey. I find it amusing and not a little instructive that nowhere in the original article does the term "executive" appear. The label "executive" has apparently been applied only in subsequent discussions of the experiment. Obviously someone with a preconceived notion of the relationship between executive activity and stress chose the term.*

Some *scientific* support for the notion of executive vulnerability can be found in a report by C. A. D'Alonzo and his coworkers from the Medical Division of E. I. du Pont de Nemours and Company on the state of health of their employees during the years from 1939 to 1953. Peptic ulcer was the only disorder found to be more common in executive personnel, and this held true for people fifty years and older. Unfortunately, the researchers didn't differentiate between gastric and duodenal ulcers.

It's become practically axiomatic among laymen and among many physicians as well that executives are more prone to ulcers than are, for example, blue-collar workers and other wage earners. But in parts of Africa, India and the Orient, farmers, other agricultural workers and unskilled laborers have a high incidence of ulcer, whereas in the industrialized nations these kinds of work are frequently associated with a low incidence. Other data suggest that white-collar workers, civil servants, small businessmen and transport workers (bus drivers, truck drivers, taxi drivers, train engineers and airline personnel) have a higher than normal tendency to develop ulcers. In still other investigations some professional groups—surgeons, business executives, military personnel of an executive rank, military pilots, overseers, managers, foremen and craftsmen—have been shown to be ulcer-prone.

You can see that there is absolutely no consistent relationship to be found between a specific occupation and the likelihood of developing ulcers. Part of the problem may stem

---

* In an attempt to track down the tag "executive," as applied to these now-celebrated monkeys, I corresponded with and subsequently spoke to Dr. Porter. Neither he nor his colleagues are certain how the term came to be used. He believes that it may have been taken from an article published in the lay literature, although none of us have been able to find it.

from the fact that many of these studies don't differentiate between gastric and duodenal ulcer.

Somewhat more convincing support for the idea that occupational factors may be important in the development of ulcers *provided a distinction is made between gastric and duodenal ulcer* comes from a study by R. Doll and F. Avery-Jones in England. They found a disproportionately large number of ulcer sufferers among foremen and business executives, while disproportionately few agricultural workers had ulcers. The high frequency of ulcers in the upper-echelon employees was found to be almost entirely due to cases of duodenal rather than gastric ulcers. Comparable observations have been made in Holland and the United States as well.

Take, for example, the case of Sverre, who seems to be typical of the kind of person who is gastric ulcer-prone. His story is based on cases reported by the Norwegian investigator K. Schanke.

VESTERÅLEN, NORWAY. 6:00 A.M., FEBRUARY 6, 1943

Sverre is a fifty-four-year-old Norwegian commercial fisherman. He's trying to eat a breakfast of fish and liver in the galley of a rolling skiff in heavy seas off the coast of the Vesterålen Islands north of the Arctic Circle. The meal is important. He may not eat again for ten to twelve hours, and his workday may last for another twenty to twenty-four hours, especially if the day's catch is a good one. During many twenty-hour workdays he gets to eat only twice.

A strong, vigorous man, he fishes for about five of the winter months, and works his small farm in Vesterålen for the rest of the year. Not given to complaints, he tends to be cheerful and complacent. Quiet and thoughtful, he seems somewhat stolid and slow in his movements. Although he has a strong belief in authority, he has very little respect for rules and regulations.

Not particularly ambitious, he's quite satisfied with his

life, accepting things as they are. He hardly personifies the stereotype of an "ulcer personality." Nevertheless, he has a gastric ulcer and has had one since age forty-seven.

He has been fishing and farming for most of his life. His first bout with stomach ulcer occurred seven winters ago during the Lofoten fishing season. When he returned to the farm, his symptoms disappeared and did not recur until the next year, again during the fishing season. He's had only occasional flare-ups during periods of heavy farmwork. The onset of his symptoms is obviously related to the great irregularity of his work and eating habits during the fishing seasons.

He'll soon stop fishing entirely, the flare-up of his ulcer being the primary cause, and spend the rest of his life in rural farming and forestry. Except for occasional periods during heavy harvest or woodcutting times, his ulcer will never again be a serious problem.

The story of Manuelo is more typical of the person with duodenal ulcer.

MIAMI, FLORIDA. 4:30 P.M., NOVEMBER 14, 1975

Manuelo is a bright, ambitious twenty-six-year-old who has been a cabdriver for five years. Manuelo was born in Cuba, but his father, a prosperous businessman, was driven from the island early in the Castro regime; he brought his wife, Manuelo and two daughters to Miami, leaving virtually all their worldly goods behind. Manuelo's father died shortly after his arrival in the United States, but he imbued his family with ambition and a strong work ethic.

Married and the father of three small children, Manuelo is in the tenth hour of his workday. He and his brother-in-law hope to build a fleet of taxis, but for the moment they are struggling to accumulate sufficient capital. Manuelo puts in twelve to sixteen hours a day, earning up to $125.00 before expenses each shift. He's extremely tense, anxious and goal-oriented.

His eating habits are about what you would expect from

someone with such a crowded schedule. He smokes two packs of cigarettes a day, drinks lots of coffee and an occasional glass of wine, and takes no aspirin. He keeps a bottle of antacids in the glove compartment of his cab and pops two tablets every two to six hours. Manny has a duodenal ulcer and has had one for two years.

The pain has increased in intensity over the past two months, and freedom from symptoms is rare. Lately he's had back pain and night pain as well. He knows his life style is "ruining" his stomach, but he's trapped until the loan for the taxi and license is paid off and his dream of a fleet can be realized.

Within six months Manuelo will be hospitalized for treatment of internal hemorrhaging. He'll ultimately undergo surgery.

These case histories reveal some of the subtle differences between those people who seem to be more likely to develop gastric ulcers and those who will tend to develop duodenal ones. The characterizations are not far-fetched and sit well with the information we have at hand. Vernon's rather colorful story may be even more convincing.

O'HARE AIRPORT. FEBRUARY 22, 1970

Vernon's a thirty-two-year-old white male who for six years has worked as an air traffic controller at one of the busiest airports in the world. He's basically healthy except for recurring mild upper mid-abdominal pain that has bothered him intermittently for three years. The pain is easily relieved by food or milk, and he's never sought medical attention for it. He smokes two and a half packs of cigarettes a day and consumes up to twenty cups of coffee, most of them during his work hours. A fifth of Scotch lasts him a month. He takes no drugs or medications of any kind except for an occasional aspirin. Highly intelligent and conscientious, he is divorced and lives alone.

He's been on duty for three hours. Fifteen minutes ago,

he almost caused a midair collision between two planes carrying a total of 270 people. The incident has understandably raised his level of anxiety sky-high. Although he is due for a meal break, he's lost his appetite. He'll be irritable for several days and suffer sleeplessness for the rest of the week. But for the moment he is trapped at his radarscope, forced to continue issuing cool, concise commands into a microphone.

In March 1970, R. R. Grayson, an internist in St. Charles, Illinois, had an unusual opportunity to study a group of people with symptoms related to chronic stress. As a result of a serious labor-management dispute between the Federal Aviation Authority and its employees, air traffic controllers in the Chicago area, in part to protest working conditions, stopped work in a "sick-out." One hundred and eleven of these men were examined over a one-year period beginning with the onset of the strike.

Eighty-six of the one hundred and eleven men examined had symptoms consistent with peptic ulcer, and all the men were further examined by barium upper-gastrointestinal x-rays. A mind-boggling 32.5 percent of the employees evaluated were shown to be suffering from previously undiagnosed and untreated ulcers. All but four had duodenal ulcer; two had combined gastric and duodenal ulcers; four had gastric ulcers alone.

I know of no other instance in which a specific occupation has been reported to have so high an association with duodenal ulcer. These observations are the most dramatic demonstration of a possible relationship between some kinds of stress and ulcers. That most of the ulcers proved to be duodenal lends further credibility to the idea that duodenal ulcers are different from gastric ulcers. While admittedly this is a relatively small sample, the extraordinary frequency of ulcers leads to one of two almost unavoidable conclusions: either there is something about being an air controller that causes duodenal ulcers, or there is something about people who are duodenal ulcer prone that makes them want to become air controllers!

While we need a more detailed analysis of similar high-risk groups, because of the many subtleties involved in the pathological process ending in duodenal ulcer, I find this report to be of much more than passing interest. Air controlling is clearly stressful and anxiety-producing.

For the moment, let's take a conservative viewpoint and conclude that the question of a cause-effect relationship between job and ulcers remains open. However, I am inclined to favor the notion that, for the duodenal variety at least, your job and the way you respond to its pressures have an important bearing on who gets ulcers and why.

5

Personality and Ulcer

The separation of psychology from the premises of biology is purely artificial, because the human psyche lives in indissoluble union with the body.

—Carl Jung (1875–1961)

The view that a peptic ulcer may be the hole in a man's stomach through which he crawls to escape from his [life]* has fairly wide acceptance.

—J. A. D. Anderson (1926–),
from "A New Look at Social Medicine"

Personality is your essential, visible character. It's what others see you to be, based on the way you act in response to them, to others, to environmental stimuli, and most impor-

---

* Anderson's original quote had "wife." I have substituted "life" partly in an effort to protect my flanks but mostly because I believe it more closely reflects the truth.

tantly, to yourself. If you like yourself it shows. If you don't, that too is apparent. Your personality represents the sum total of your physical, intellectual, emotional, social and behavioral characteristics. The nuances and subtle variations of your personality stem from genetic, interpersonal and environmental factors. Exactly when and how your personality begins to develop is still a matter of speculation.

Peptic ulcer, more than any other disorder, is thought of by lay people and physicians as being a psychosomatic disease —that is, one partly derived from psychological forces. The functions of many of the body's organs are influenced by the brain's interpretation of the stimuli constantly bombarding it. Considerable evidence links mental and emotional processes with bodily function. Rapid heartbeat and dryness of the mouth in the face of anxiety, diarrhea during stress, blushing in response to embarrassment, and crying as a reaction to sadness and depression are only a few familiar examples.

More subtle physiological and biochemical processes are also affected by emotions. For example, by-products of increased adrenal-gland secretions can be detected in the blood and urine of people subjected to certain kinds of "fight or flight" situations. Change in pituitary and thyroid function under similar conditions is still another example. Most importantly (at least from the point of view of people with ulcers), we know that a variety of mentally perceived stimuli— those which register on both a conscious and an unconscious level—can change the muscular activity of the gastrointestinal tract and, especially, the ability of the stomach to produce acid and pepsin. Pavlov's studies on dogs were among the earliest to show that the sight, taste or smell of food all caused change in stomach function.

In 1825, W. Beaumont, an Army surgeon, reported a case demonstrating a clear-cut relationship between stomach activity and conscious as well as suppressed emotional reactions. As a result of a close-range gunshot wound, Alexis St.

Martin, a rough-and-tumble Canadian trapper, developed a fistula (a permanent opening) in his abdominal wall. The fistula connected his stomach to the skin of his abdomen and allowed Beaumont to directly observe and evaluate the color, thickness and secretions of St. Martin's stomach lining. Based on these remarkable observations Beaumont reported that "in fear, anger, or whatever tones down or disturbs the nervous system, the gastric mucosa sometimes becomes red and dry, sometimes pale and moist and loses its shining, healthy appearance; the secretions are disturbed, greatly diminished or entirely inhibited."

In more recent times, other observers have had similar opportunities. In the case of a rather famous fistula patient called "Tom," researchers S. Wolf and H. G. Wolff also found the gastric lining to be responsive to emotion. They observed that during periods of anger, rage, anxiety or resentment small superficial erosions and even tiny ruptured capillaries with hemorrhage could be seen in the gastric mucosa.

The connections these pioneers made between specific emotional states and specific stomach changes may not be entirely valid, however. Unfortunately, the complexities of human emotional behavior are such that we often camouflage our true feelings. Subtle variations in *sub*conscious emotional activity could have been entirely missed or wrongly construed by the observers.

A colorful modern observation showing a relationship between gastric-acid production and a particular form of stress was related by my friend Ed Storer.*

A lawyer who had been hospitalized for treatment of a duodenal ulcer and who fancied himself as quite a chess player was challenged to a game by [the late] Dr. James S. Clarke.

* In *The Physiology and Treatment of Peptic Ulcer*. Chicago: University of Chicago Press.

After [a stomach tube] was placed into the fasting patient's stomach and connected to suction, Clarke proceeded to frustrate him in a game of chess; the patient was beaten rather badly. As the tension mounted in the game, so, too, did the gastric secretion mount as measured by the rate of accumulation of gastric content in the collecting bottle. His resentment and the over-secretion of acid apparently lasted for some hours [it roughly doubled on the night of the chess game, falling back again to half that on the following night].

Studies on the production of stomach acid in male college students show that these men secrete significantly more gastric acid during examination periods than during periods in which no exams were given. G. F. Mahl and his coworkers concluded that the rise in stomach acid correlated very closely with the degree of anxiety shown by the subject. It was inferred that anxiety causes increased acid secretion. Since acid is known to be fundamental in causing ulcers, they reasoned that anxiety may well be an underlying factor.

While organic disease and emotional disturbances often exist simultaneously, this is no proof of a cause-and-effect relationship. Still, this hasn't prevented many of us from developing a preconceived idea of what the "typical" person with ulcers is like. "He's an ulcer type" is a common expression.

Based on what we currently know about ulcers and personality, these generalizations are about as useful as equating long hair and jeans with being a hippie. Nevertheless, personality characteristics commonly associated with people with ulcers are ambitiousness, conscientiousness, drive, nervousness, anxiety, worry, instability, insecurity, restlessness, and so on. R. S. Paffenbarger of the California State Department of Health and his group have expressed the problem of relating personality and ulcer rather well: "The general image of a likely subject for peptic ulcer is an inveterate coffee drinker and cigarette smoker, employed in a sedentary but stressful occupation, fearful of failure and relieving his tensions by overindulgence in alcohol. *Unclear is whether this pattern is predictive of ulcer or the ulcer is productive of the pattern.* (Emphasis mine)"

There is nothing like complete agreement on which personality characteristics are consistently identifiable in the disorder. In fact, in the cases of subjects with a fistula, various observations of the stomach's *anatomic* and *physiological* responses to the same emotion don't jibe. Fear and anger caused redness of the mucosa and small hemorrhages in the stomachs of some of these subjects, as well as an increase in the concentration of acid in the gastric juice. In other subjects, however, an increase in the volume of acid and pepsin was observed during periods of *contentment.*

These contradictory findings emphasize that either there are marked variations in stomach response to the same state of mind or that the patient's true state of mind is subject to error in interpretation. At the very best, these discrepancies may be based on the imperfect and primitive nature of the techniques used for observation. At worst, they suggest that consistent patterns of response to specific emotions have not yet been convincingly shown.

I don't doubt that there is a link between the stomach and the mind; most of us who have studied the phenomenon feel that the connection is real. At least one study reported by T. Szasz and his coworkers suggests that the bond is based on nervous pathways rather than on hormonal or biochemical routes. Unfortunately, the data come from only one patient, in whom it was noted that open hostility caused a rise in gastric-acid secretion. Following this observation, the patient underwent an operation in which the vagus nerves were cut. Once the nervous pathway was interrupted, psychic stress no longer stimulated acid.

This kind of observation has led surgeons to conclude that whatever the true effect of emotion on gastric secretion, it is mediated by way of the vagus nerves. Widespread confidence in this idea is one of the bases of all modern surgery for people with ulcers (see Chapter 14).

Most articles on the relationship between personality and the development of ulcers that have appeared in the scientific literature over the last forty-five years pay homage to the beautifully constructed and well thought out concepts advocated by the psychoanalyst F. Alexander in 1934. He postulated that a specific *conflict* in a person's life rather than a specific personality type was the essence of the causation of peptic ulcers. His work has been quoted, misquoted, extended and modified. His original theories are immensely significant, not only because they may be close to the truth, but because they have influenced so much of the thought on the subject.

Alexander believed that ulcer-prone people are oral-dependent and passive in situations where more active and open aggression is more appropriate. In somewhat simpler terms, ulcers may be caused by a kind of inner-directed hostility or discontent stemming from a strong childish need to be looked after and loved, a need that may be rejected or denied. One interpretation of Alexander's view is to equate milk (typically recommended in ulcer diets) with motherly love; the very existence of the ulcer allows the patient to be cared for and "mothered" in a way acceptable to both the patient and society.

Distinguished scientists H. Shay and D. C. H. Sun have verbalized Alexander's ideas in another way. They feel that a typical ulcer-prone person thinks of himself as efficient, active, and productive: "I give to everybody, help people, assume responsibility, like to have people depend upon me, like to be the effective leader and the self-sufficient, and I have an active or even aggressive personality." However, Shay and Sun found "in the unconscious exactly the opposite attitude, an extreme violent craving for love and the need for dependence and help. These tendencies . . . are repressed and denied by the patient and associated with violent conflicts."

These concepts have been endorsed, in part because they "fit" the popular notion. H. M. Spiro has written that "most physicians will agree with, and the popular press will support . . . [that] ulcer patients as a group tend to repress their emotions or tend to at least inhibit outward expressions of strongly held feelings. The duodenal ulcer patient seems to have learned at a very early age to prefer to keep peace rather than to flail out with his hands or his tongue." In other words, ulcer patients seem to "anger-in."

Under experimental laboratory conditions, when the cortex of the brain is stimulated by either electrical or chemical means, changes in the stomach's muscular activity, blood flow and ability to make acid have been observed. Environmental events—even those not consciously noticed—do influence the individual. Freud and Jung postulated that these events are capable of starting a chain reaction in which emotions, muscular activity and body organ function, as well as general behavior, may be affected.

Another modification of Alexander's conflict theory has been proposed by G. L. Engel, a psychiatrist who supports the notion of a powerful relationship between emotional and psychological processes and the function of the stomach. He believes that the newborn infant's cycle of hunger and satisfaction (relief of hunger) is a basic biological influence. To him, this represents the primary establishment of an "oral" type of association between mother and child; if it prospers, it is mutually gratifying. If it doesn't succeed, it may form the basis for discord and dissatisfaction for both the infant and the mother.

Engel characterizes ulcer-prone people as "oral dependent"—more apt to suck, mouth and chew gum, pencils, pipes, cigarettes and cigars, knuckles and fingernails. Oral orientation may be expressed by the use of such terms of endearment and pleasure as "how sweet" and "I could eat you up," or of displeasure (distaste!) as "You make me sick (to my stomach)."

Most significantly, however, Engel endorses the commonly held idea that there are indeed identifiable ulcer personality types. Based on his own observations as well as those of others, he describes three.

THE PSEUDO-INDEPENDENT

Pseudo-independent people typically deny their feelings of dependency and present themselves as strong, independent types. They're viewed as self-reliant, aggressive and controlling, although this may in fact be illusory. Men of this type are super-macho, while pseudo-independent women may exhibit stereotypically masculine characteristics. Pseudo-independents belittle those who express the need for rest and relaxation or vacations; they look down upon those whom they consider weak and dependent. In our own society these characteristics are often identified with success.

Engel sees them as controlling, dominant types inclined to coerce others into providing for their needs. "In this manner they can maintain, at an unconscious level, gratification of their true dependent requirements. The spouse, for example, is most likely to be the long-suffering self-denying provider, while the patients see themselves as powerful and self-sufficient."

An example of such a person, based on my own experience, is Lewis.

LOS ANGELES, CALIFORNIA. 10:01 A.M., JANUARY 28, 1977

Lewis is the fifty-nine-year-old chief executive officer of a thriving advertising agency, a position he assumed when the highly respected and revered founder of the company reached mandatory retirement age. A former star college athlete, he's five feet eight inches tall, weighs two hundred pounds, and is getting bald.

He's about to chair a meeting of the executive committee, and his subordinates are not looking forward to it. Disliked for his autocratic, domineering and manipulative ways, he's a mixture of slightly above average competence and an exaggerated conception of his own abilities. Good at organization of personnel and delegation of authority, he has limited creativity and imagination in a field where both are prized.

He's widely regarded as selfish, stubborn, and demanding. Fond of coarse jokes and loud dress, he's prone to braggadocio, particularly about his sexual exploits and physical prowess (largely discounted as fantasy by his embarrassed listeners). But in an unguarded moment he has been heard to say that he can't make it with straight women and prefers prostitutes. Married and divorced three times, he currently lives alone.

At least two of the committee members will be mildly put out by his petty humiliations and cheap shots, and although votes will be taken on various issues, no one doubts that the "democratic process" is only a façade. All decisions will be made by him and him alone.

Lew has had an ulcer since a year after he took his current job. There have been no complications, but symptoms are fairly unremitting and continuous throughout the year.

THE PASSIVE DEPENDENT

In this type, according to Engel, the dependent needs are expressed openly and exist on the conscious level as well. Compliant, passive, ingratiating, eager to please, these people are also jealous, clinging, possessive and dependent. Passive-dependent men may display what are commonly termed effeminate traits.

Rae-Ellen typifies the passive-dependent ulcer-prone woman.

WASHINGTON, D.C. 7:15 A.M., JUNE 16, 1975

Rae-Ellen is an attractive twenty-three-year-old nurse. She's about to go off duty after having worked two consecutive eight-hour shifts—her own plus that of her close friend Marie who had a "heavy weekend date" and asked Rae-Ellen to substitute for her. Friendly, warm and always willing, Rae-Ellen agreed to do so, although it means almost sixteen straight hours on her feet. She wants to be liked; in fact she wants to be loved.

Her relationships with men haven't been terribly successful. She has been passed from man to man ever since age seventeen, but she seems to turn them off after a while, despite her submissiveness, because of her dependent, clinging and demanding ways. Her latest affair is a disaster; yet she can't break with him, even though he has used her sexually, socially and professionally.

For the past six weeks she's been dieting intensively. She smokes a pack and a half a day and drinks a cocktail or two after work and wine with dinner.

The pain in her upper mid-abdomen penetrates through to her back, is only partially relieved by food and has been costing her sleep. Her face is drawn, and heavy lines are developing under her eyes. She has sought medical advice, and on the basis of her history alone has been told she has an ulcer.

She hasn't been able to modify her smoking, drinking, eating and work habits, nor has she been able to break up with her current male friend. However, she does take antacids regularly, with moderate to good relief of symptoms. She'll soon seek more competent medical advice and a thorough evaluation. X-rays will reveal a typical chronic duodenal ulcer, and a rather extensive reorganization of her life will be advised. She'll try to comply by working regular shifts only, modifying her dietary habits, cutting down on drinking and smoking, and getting more rest. Although she'll never be operated on, her ulcer will plague her off and on for the rest of her life.

THE ACTING OUT

Engel sees this group as satisfying their dependent needs by an immature demanding personality ("I want what I want when I want it"). They commonly disregard the needs and rights of others and may even resort to sociopathic or criminal acts to get their own way. They are the drifters, the chronically unemployed, the irresponsible members of society. They are often addicted to drugs, tobacco or alcohol, and tend to be inconsiderate and parasitic in their personal relationships.

William is another example from my own experience.

BOSTON, MASSACHUSETTS. 4:52 P.M., DECEMBER 15, 1972

William is twenty-six-years-old. He's lying in his sleeping bag on the floor of the shabby apartment he shares with three other men and two women. He has been vomiting for three days, his abdomen is concave, and he can't hold any food down. Two of his friends will take him to the hospital, where he'll be admitted for gastric retention and an obstructing duodenal ulcer.

Willie is the product of a middle-class suburban family. His school work was average, and he graduated without any particular distinction and without training for any specific line of work. He's had a series of menial jobs—bus boy, gasstation attendant, and so forth—but rarely works longer than a few months. Either he tires of the job or he's asked to leave.

Alternately cocky and sullen, he's demanding in his relationships with others, borrows money often but rarely repays it, and will take what he wants if it's not given to him. He smokes pot heavily, drinks alcohol when it's available, and regularly uses uppers for a quick high. He takes what he can and gives as little as possible in return.

After several days of stomach suction and restoration of his body fluids by intravenous infusions, he'll be operated on. Although his postoperative course will be uncomplicated, he'll revisit the hospital many times for evaluation of vague abdominal complaints, the precise cause of which will never be determined.

These are clearly defined personality categories—no hedging here. Many, though by no means all, of the people with peptic ulcers with whom I've dealt over the years can be neatly placed into one of them, and I can sense many readers saying, "He's right! I *know* people with ulcers who are like that. Or I *am* like that!"

One disturbing aspect of such neat categorizations is that they involve very common personality characteristics. Of the many people who fit one or another of these descriptions, some will have an ulcer and some won't. Certainly not all people suffering from ulcers will fit neatly into Engel's three categories. Conversely, not every person who matches one of the descriptions has or will develop ulcers.

By labeling his concept "somatopsychic-psychosomatic," Engel intends to convey that the body processes responsible for ulcer development (by increased acid secretion, for example), are also contributory to the development of specific personality and psychological characteristics. But are these personality traits significantly more characteristic of the ulcer-prone person than of the population at large?

Some studies suggest that they are. In one, reported by M. H. Alp, J. H. Court and K. A. Grant of the University of Adelaide, 181 South Australians with a past history of chronic stomach ulcers were observed. It was concluded that these people shared three personality traits: all were highly anxious, submissive with a strong tendency to develop depression, and tough-minded. "Tough-mindedness" was defined as an aggressive, no-nonsense, self-sufficient approach to things. The authors acknowledged, however, that since they studied patients who had already developed ulcers, they couldn't determine whether the ulcer caused the attitudes or the attitudes were basic to the development of the ulcers. They also noted that, when compared with age- and sex-matched persons without a history of stomach ulcers, these people were under greater domestic and financial stress, and that they consumed more aspirin, alcohol and cigarettes.

Finally, and perhaps most interestingly, although persons with chronic stomach ulcers were characteristically independent and self-sufficient, they were, somewhat paradoxically, especially prone to periods of anxiety and depression. These studies suggest that internal conflicts between what you are sexually and how you act or want to act, coupled with a poor ability to express aggression ("anger-out"), may be significant in causing ulcers.

Studies of twins offer an unusual opportunity to compare the effects of hereditary, environmental and psychological factors. Identical twins separated at birth or during early childhood are presumably hereditarily identical, while the environments in which they grow up differ. Conversely, identical twins who grow up together have virtually identical or very similar genetic and environmental backgrounds.

If *only one of a pair of identical twins has an ulcer,* or if one develops an ulcer far in advance of the other, we should be able to detect pertinent personality or conflict mechanisms associated with the development of the disorder. Consider the case of Jason and Jacques.

NEWARK, NEW JERSEY. JULY 15, 1967

Jason and Jacques are thirty-seven-year-old identical twins, practicing pharmacists who operate a thriving drugstore concession in a major department store chain. Brought up in a warm and loving middle-class family, they've been close all of their lives. Both bachelors, they work and live together.

Jason is the "dominant" twin, as they both agree, and is

more independent, self-assertive and outgoing. Jacques is quieter and more compliant; he tends to look to his brother before making even relatively minor decisions or commitments. They get along very well.

Their lives are about to change. Their elderly parents, who also lived in Newark and for whom the boys provided total support, have both just died within weeks of each other, a not uncommon phenomenon. Jason is depressed, but within three months he will have regained his usual cheerful and outgoing manner. Not so Jacques. Shortly after his father's funeral he began to notice occasional "hunger pains." They have gradually become more severe, and within three months his doctor will document a full-blown duodenal ulcer.

To date, Jason remains well. Jacques is well, too, but in 1972 he underwent surgery for his ulcer, which couldn't be controlled by medication.

G. Eberhard, a Scandinavian investigator, studied the personalities of thirty pairs of identical twins in which at least one twin had an ulcer. He found that the twin with an ulcer was significantly more sensitive to stress, and that nervous complaints were observed more frequently in the twin with ulcers than in the healthy twin. He concluded that since both twins had been exposed to the same amount of stress growing up, the twin who developed an ulcer had an impaired emotional defense mechanism when compared to the twin without one, or to the twin with a later onset of ulcer. The higher frequency of nervous complaints in the twins with ulcers was thought to be related to an increase in sensitivity to stress—that is, *to a more intense interpretation of the environment as stressful*—since both twins were judged to have been exposed to the same degree of stressful trauma.

In an article published in 1975 in the prestigious journal *Gastroenterology,* a distinguished group of physicians and students of peptic ulcer concluded that short-term gastrointestinal disturbances may be related to psychosomatic forces.

But they agreed that for long-term disorders such as duodenal ulcer, the conclusions are somewhat less certain.

A second question that must be answered before we can
link a specific personality type with ulcers is: Can we predict *in advance* which segment of the population is prone to
the development of ulcers and which is not? H. Weiner,
I. A. Mirsky and their associates succeeded in accomplishing
such a feat. In a now-classic study carried out in 1957, they
predicted, using Alexander's hypothesis of personality and
conflict in the cause of ulcers, which newly inducted Army
recruits would develop ulcers during the stress of basic military training. The experiment deserves acclaim not only
for its innovative and imaginative spirit but also for its close
adherence to restrictive scientific principles. In the twenty
years since its completion, no one has been able to improve
on it.

The research team began with the prediction that duodenal ulcers *should* develop when an individual with a high
sustained output of stomach acid is exposed to a particular
environmental situation capable of triggering a "psychic"
conflict and of inducing "psychic" tension. The team's theory
was that when physiological, psychological and social factors
are all brought to bear simultaneously on an individual, they
should join together to produce peptic ulcer.

Two thousand seventy-three Army draftees being proc-
essed at an induction camp were studied. Using blood studies
to determine the level of pepsinogen produced, the researchers selected a group of sixty-three over-secretors and one of
fifty-seven under-secretors. All of these men underwent complete gastrointestinal x-ray studies and various psychological
examinations. They were then sent to the basic training area.
All but thirteen of the original group were again given psychological and x-ray testing some time between the eighth
and sixteenth week of their basic training.

The first x-ray examination picked up four patients with
evidence of ulcers, all of whom came from the group of

over-secretors. One became a disciplinary problem and was subsequently confined to the stockade; another went AWOL; a third completed basic training without incident; the fourth was discharged from the service because of the active ulcer.

At the time of the second x-ray examination, after basic training was well under way, five more men who'd had no signs of ulcer problems at the beginning of the study were found to have an active ulcer. All of the subjects who initially had or who subsequently developed duodenal ulcers came from the over-secretor group. Furthermore, if only the top 5 percent of these over-secretors was considered, *an additional* nine men developed duodenal ulcers during a relatively brief interval. These are extraordinary findings—while under a special kind of stress a group predicted to be ulcer-prone actually developed ulcers.

In a second, much longer term study of a population of 1,600 children several months to sixteen years old and 4,460 adults, Mirsky selected out, as an over-secreting group, the 2 percent with the highest concentration of blood pepsinogen levels, and the 2 percent with the lowest concentration of pepsinogen. Although no specific data were reported and the study was still in progress at the time it was published, "a fairly large number of healthy over-secretors who have been followed for several years developed the typical signs and symptoms of duodenal ulcer which was subsequently proven by x-ray. In contrast, none of the individuals comprising the under-secretor group developed the ulcer syndrome." An unexpectedly high incidence of duodenal ulcer was found in the 2 percent of children with the highest serum pepsinogen concentrations. About one in ten developed duodenal ulcers.

Finally, and perhaps most importantly from the point of view of evaluating personality as a factor in the development of ulcers, both the short- and long-term studies revealed that the over-secretors who *never* developed ulcers seemed to exhibit essentially the same personality structure and the same psychodynamic pattern described by Alexander in 1934. These people showed intense, primarily oral needs, which were acted out in terms of a wish to be fed, to depend upon others and to seek close bodily contact. Excessive drinking, gambling, delinquency and promiscuity were seen in this group too.

Those Army recruits who developed ulcers differed from the over-secretors who did not develop ulcers *only* in the intensity in which they attempted to develop or sustain relationships with other men. They demonstrated anxiety and a fear of expressing hostility ("anger-in"). They went to extremes to rationalize, deny or subdue these feelings. The need to please their superior officers was particularly noteworthy.

Mirsky has concluded that some valid and convincing inferences can be drawn from these very complex observations. Thus, in his view, the actual development of an ulcer would seem to result from the combination of at least three basic factors: a) the overproduction of acid gastric juice; b) a specific personality type; c) an environmentally stressful situation that acts as a catalyst. When all three of these factors are brought to bear on an individual, the net result *may* be peptic ulcer.

Mirsky clarifies his analysis by stating that "those who insist that the development of duodenal ulcer is determined solely by 'organic' factors are as fallacious as those who claim that 'psychic' factors are the sole determinants." And elsewhere: "neither a high rate of gastric secretion nor a specific psychodynamic constellation is independently responsible for the development of peptic ulcer."

Those of us trained in biological disciplines tend to be skeptical of ideas not fully supported by solid scientific evidence. It isn't proven that personality traits and/or conflicts contribute significantly to the cause of ulcers. It *is* an attractive probability. The burden of proof rests with those who question this.

6

Coffee, Tea, Tobacco, Alcohol and Aspirin

How to Stay Young

1) Avoid fried meats which angry up the blood.
2) If your stomach disputes you, lie down and pacify it with cool thoughts.
3) Keep the juices flowing by jangling around gently as you move.
4) Go very light on the vices, such as carrying on in society. The social ramble ain't restful.
5) Avoid running at all times.
6) Don't look back. Something might be gaining on you.

—Leroy (Satchel) Paige

"Life style" means so many things to different people that it almost defies definition. It has economic, political, social and sexual overtones. It reflects the options the world has thrust upon us, and it mirrors those we have picked to exercise. Life style has to do with our personal behavior patterns —the number of hours we sleep, our work schedules, the way we clean our houses and spend our money. It also refers to the drugs we take to help us relax, to relieve tension, to satisfy oral cravings and to control pain—coffee, tea, tobacco, alcohol and aspirin.

These personal habits are commonly held responsible for causing ulcers. Since great quantities of tobacco, coffee, tea, alcohol and aspirin are used throughout the Western world, it's important to give them careful consideration.

COFFEE AND TEA

Folklore has it that coffee was discovered by Abyssinian goatherds over eleven hundred years ago. They noted an unusually spirited response in their goats after the animals had eaten the berries from a wild bush. The local monks concocted a beverage from the beans and drank it to keep them awake during the long night hours of prayer.

Conflicting opinions characterized its early acceptance. Mohammed, writing in the Koran, denounced coffee as intoxicating at about the same time that Pope Clement VIII designated it a "truly Christian beverage." It gained extraordinary popularity during the period of the Renaissance and allegedly helped to inspire creativity and imagination. Voltaire, a man of sparkling wit and perceptive commentary, was an addict and is said to have consumed up to fifty cups a day. Yet it wasn't until the imposition of an intolerable tax on tea resulted in the Boston Tea Party that coffee began to attain the extraordinary popularity it enjoys today in the United States.

And coffee's popularity *is* extraordinary. Americans consume approximately 211 billion cups of coffee per year— roughly three cups per day for every man, woman and child in this country.* At 1977 prices of three dollars plus per pound, coffee is big business. It's become so much a part of the American way of life that we couldn't do without it.

We may drink coffee for its warmth, aroma and taste, but it is the caffeine in it that affects us most. Caffeine, together with some related compounds, is found not only in the coffee bean, but also in tea leaves, cocoa, and cola drinks. These contain, among other things, derivatives of cola nuts, which are about 2 percent caffeine. Theobromine, also found in cola drinks, has many of the same effects as caffeine.

The caffeine content in tea leaves is somewhat higher. A cup of tea contains about 100 to 150 milligrams, a dose sufficient to cause its pharmacologic effects. A twelve-ounce bottle of Coca-Cola contains about one-third to one-half as much caffeine as a cup of coffee.

Caffeine has some potentially desirable effects on the body. It stimulates the central nervous system, often resulting in exceptionally clear-minded thinking. It can also decrease fatigue and drowsiness and elevate mood. Caffeine makes you more sensitive to environmental stimuli, improves muscle and brain-eye-hand reflexes, and increases efficiency. Other reactions we have to caffeine include an increased flow of urine from the kidneys, a relaxation of the muscles controlling the bronchial tubes of the lungs, and a stimulation of heart muscle.

Many people know that they are more or less dependent on coffee. There are people who simply can't start their day without a cup or two of hot coffee and who may need five to fifty cups a day to sustain the heightened awareness and sharper intellectual capacity that coffee affords. But does moderate or heavy coffee drinking have an adverse effect on

* Material provided me by K. A. Anderson, director of the Coffee Information Institute, reveals that as of early 1977 the average annual worldwide coffee production amounted to about 72 million bags weighing 132 pounds each. Coffee consumption in the United States alone is estimated at between 20 and 21 million bags each year.

the gastrointestinal tract? Does it cause ulcers, retard their ability to heal, or increase the frequency of flare-ups and recurrences?

In a provocative study on this subject, R. S. Paffenbarger and his associates from the University of California and the Harvard Schools of Public Health analyzed the responses to a questionnaire by 480 former college students who developed ulcers some time after graduation. A review of college health records containing information recorded on the students *before* they developed ulcers revealed certain predisposing habits. While neither tea nor alcohol consumed during college seemed to influence the future development of peptic ulcers, the single most important predictor of ulcer was habitual coffee drinking. Interestingly enough, the more milk a person consumed during the college years, the less likely he or she was to develop ulcers in the future.

Since animal experiments have shown that caffeine increases gastric-acid secretion, it's been suggested that caffeine makes you more susceptible to peptic ulcer, or aggravates the condition. However, evidence to the contrary can be found in a study conducted at the National Naval Medical Center in Bethesda, Maryland, under the direction of R. B. Johnson. After measuring gastric-acid secretion in the unstimulated or resting stomach of healthy volunteers, Johnson and his coworkers gave these volunteers either pure caffeine or caffeine in the form of three different brands of instant coffee. The researchers found that the peak amount of gastric acid secreted by the coffee drinkers and by those who were given pure caffeine didn't vary significantly from acid measured during the unstimulated state. They concluded that, although coffee drinking causes a slight increase in acid, moderate consumption of coffee will probably not adversely affect ulcers.

Isolating the effects of coffee from those of other factors is difficult because people who drink a lot of coffee tend to smoke cigarettes and drink alcohol (which is also an acid stimulant) as well. Possibly the *kind* of person who depends on coffee, alcohol and tobacco is also ulcer-prone. Thus proving that caffeine has a role in the causation or retarded healing of ulcers is difficult.

Although caffeine is clearly a gastric-acid stimulant and has been used for the activation of stomach juices in laboratory animals for many years, there are few grounds for believing that moderate amounts of coffee, tea or cola have any adverse effects on the natural history of peptic ulcers. An article in the *New York Medical Journal and Medical Record* of April 18, 1923, outlines one approach:

> This whole question has been exaggerated. Coffee in moderation does not produce . . . ailments. Removal of the coffee from the diet does not cure them. . . . It would be well to look at the coffee question squarely and not cover this situation by inane avoidances. Coffee is one of the mainstays of our rapid civilization. Those adults who wish to live and enjoy life, let them drink their coffee in peace. Those who wish to ascribe illness or nervousness to magical causes, let them abandon it.

TOBACCO SMOKING

If coffee is big business in the United States, tobacco is bigger. According to the latest data available, in 1975 Americans spent almost $15.6 billion (a record high) on tobacco and tobacco products. As a nation we smoke approximately 2.5 cigarettes for every cup of coffee we drink. We "consume" 5.8 billion cigars, 52.6 million pounds of pipe and roll-your-own tobacco, 79.1 million pounds of chewing tobacco and 25.3 million pounds of snuff each year.

Smoking tobacco is undoubtedly hazardous to your health. We know that it shortens life on the average by at least five years. The adverse effects of smoking on the heart, lungs and other organ systems are clearly documented. In fact, if the kind of data indicting tobacco as a health hazard were applied to some other commodity—say, for example, rutabaga—everyone would undoubtedly stop eating rutabaga. There is something that makes tobacco different.

The psychological dependence most smokers build up on tobacco smoking and their inability to give it up puts it in the category of compulsive drug use. As with coffee, the taste, aroma, warmth and oral satisfaction involved in smoking tobacco may account, in large measure, for its widespread use. The nicotine content of tobacco and its effect on our systems is undoubtedly of equal importance.

We know of no therapeutic use for the drug nicotine. From a medical point of view, therefore, it's chiefly of interest for its toxic features. Nicotine has a profound stimulatory effect on the central nervous system. It can produce, in appropriate doses, both tremors and convulsions. It can stimulate respiration and cause nausea and vomiting; unlike caffeine, it slows the urine-producing action of the kidneys.

We're primarily concerned with the effect of nicotine on the gastrointestinal tract. While it can stimulate the intestine enough to cause diarrhea, this effect, depending upon the dose, is usually followed by a decrease in the muscular activity of the bowel. So-called hunger contractions seem to be reflexively abolished by the smoking of as little as one cigarette, and this depressive effect may last as long as an hour. The time it takes the stomach to empty its contents doesn't seem to be significantly altered by heavy smoking, but the actual amount of acid secreted by the stomach may be reduced. Both the volume and the concentration of acid in the fasting or unstimulated stomach appear to be decreased in many normal subjects as well as in people with ulcers.

Controlled studies have produced only weak and unconvincing evidence for a cause-and-effect relationship between smoking and peptic ulcer. In fact, in light of what we know of the physiologic action of nicotine on the gastrointestinal tract, a case could easily be made that patients with peptic ulcer smoke because it actually makes them feel better. Yet studies showing that smoking is bad for people with ulcers are not hard to come by. Some sources have indicated that smokers who inhale have a much higher rate of duodenal ulcer than a control population of smokers who don't. Other studies have purported to show that quitting cigarette smoking encourages the healing of ulcers, but that simply cutting down does not.

Studies carried out in England have shown that more patients with gastric ulcers smoked than patients without ulcers or patients with duodenal ulcers. The authors weren't able to determine a relationship between the amount of tobacco smoked and the development of either gastric or duodenal ulcer. But they suggested that if smoking was *completely* stopped, gastric ulcers did heal faster. They concluded that smoking *is* in fact causally related to peptic ulcer.

From other studies we know that there's an increase in the death rate from peptic ulcer in patients who smoke. However, this could be related to such other bad effects of smoking as the damage it does to the lungs and the heart. Paradoxically, the mortality rate has been shown to be highest among moderate or light smokers, not among heavy smokers. Still other studies have shown a significantly higher than normal risk of early death in patients with gastric ulcers who are cigar, pipe and cigarette smokers.

In groups of patients with complications of duodenal ulcer, there seem to be an inordinately large number of cigarette smokers. Duodenal ulcer patients who smoke usually began at an earlier age.

In a study of the relationship between gastric acid secretion body habits, blood groups, smoking and the ultimate development of ulcer, B. H. Novis and his coworkers found that the unstimulated output of acid was positively related to the number of cigarettes smoked per day. They speculated that cigarette smoking over a long period of time stimulated either the vagus nerves or the production of the hormone gastrin.

R. R. Monson did a particularly fine study of the relationship between cigarette smoking, body form and peptic ulcer in physicians with gastric or duodenal ulcers. Physicians are presumably more capable of giving precise and reliable information on the absence or presence of ulcer and on their smoking, alcohol or coffee habits. Monson concluded that while there is an association between smoking and peptic ulcer, this is not necessarily cause and effect. In fact, there was very little evidence that smoking causes peptic ulcer or adversely affects the healing of ulcer *"through the medium of gastric secretory changes."*

Ulcers are more common in smokers, but it may be, as I have pointed out before, that whatever causes a person to smoke may also be important in the future development of ulcers. Smoking and ulcers, while related in incidence, may be dependent upon a third as-yet-unknown factor. As a group, smokers may differ from nonsmokers in both physical constitution and personality. For example, studies comparing smokers and nonsmokers have shown that among men who smoke, over one-third drink six cups of coffee per day. Only one in twelve nonsmokers drink that much coffee. Ninety percent of male smokers drink alcohol, as compared to only 75 percent of nonsmokers. While peptic ulcer is found twice as often in smokers as in nonsmokers, the same relationship holds true for people who drink more than six cups of coffee per day.

Much of the data published on the effect of tobacco smoking and coffee on peptic ulcer indicates that no clear-cut conclusions can be drawn. While caffeine *is* a stimulant of gastric secretion, nicotine probably is not. Neither habit, at least in moderation, has any lasting or important effect on ulcer symptoms, the occurrence of ulcers, or the rate at which ulcers heal.

Many physicians maintain that the chronic peptic ulcer patient should avoid both coffee and tobacco, but I don't ask patients to give them up completely in the periods between attacks. In fact, it's been my impression that if a doctor is too adamant in his control of these habits, the restrictions in and of themselves may have an adverse effect. It seems sensible, in light of the information we have available to us on the specific pharmacologic and physiologic effects of nicotine and caffeine, to advise people with ulcers to use both in moderation, if they must use them at all.

Certainly the evidence for smoking's effect on other organ systems is both persuasive and conclusive: smoking is extremely hazardous to health and will shorten life. But with regard to ulcers, complete elimination of drinking coffee and smoking based on what we now know is inappropriate. "Moderation in all things—and especially in moderation itself."

ALCOHOL

An alcoholic has been waggishly defined as a person who drinks more than his doctor. For some, two drinks per day on a regular basis constitute an alcoholic habit. Some alcoholics never drink hard liquor, only wine or beer. While it's possible to measure the amount of alcohol in each drink, it's very difficult to define alcoholism in terms of the amount of alcohol consumed.

Alcohol is also very important economically to the American people. Based on information from the 1976 *Liquor Handbook*, we spent an estimated $13,908,000,000 on distilled spirits, $2,856,000,000 on wine and $15,832,000,000 on beer in the year 1975. We actually drank 1.98 gallons of whiskey, 1.70 gallons of wine and 21.6 gallons of beer for every man, woman and child. We are a nation awash in alcohol.

Alcohol has a direct pharmacologic effect on the gastro-intestinal tract and is capable of causing ulcerations. The way in which alcohol stimulates gastric-acid secretion seems complex. In animals alcohol causes the release of gastrin, a stimulant of gastric secretion, from the antrum, the primary source of gastrin. But in humans, it's been difficult to show an increase in blood levels of gastrin after drinking. Alcohol given intravenously increases acid secretion in animals whose antrum has been removed. This suggests that alcohol may have a direct effect on the acid-secreting cells of the stomach, without the need for release of gastrin as an intermediary factor. Alcohol *does* intensify the effect of caffeine on gastric secretion, so it may enhance the production of acid when both alcohol and coffee are consumed at the same time, or in close relation to each other.

We know, too, that the direct application of alcohol to the lining of the stomach can cause cell-wall disruption. Once this barrier is broken, acid may actually "leak back" into the cells, exaggerating tissue damage. Most heavy users of alcohol have a condition known as chronic gastritis, or an in-flammation of the gastric mucosa. Even in a nonalcoholic, large amounts of highly concentrated alcohol can cause a similar inflammation. But there is no evidence that people with gastritis are *more* susceptible to ulcers, and gastritis may simply be another form of chronic stomach inflamma-tion, not specifically related to ulcers.

One way to gain some insight into the possible connection between alcohol and ulcers is to look for a correlation be-tween the frequency of ulcers and the amount people drink. For example, R. R. Grayson investigated the incidence of peptic ulcer in almost 1,000 problem drinkers who worked for a large American corporation employing over 100,000 people. Ulcer disease was twice as common among those who drank to excess as among a group of matched controls. Three percent of the problem drinkers were known to have gastric ulcers, and 8 percent had duodenal ulcers. However, these figures aren't greatly at variance with the normal distribution of ulcer in the nondrinking population. In a different study from Sweden, a high consumption of alcohol by Army trainees during basic military preparation was found to be associated with a predisposition to emotional difficulties and problems in adaptation, but *not* with the development of ulcers.

In an interesting analysis of the effects of tobacco, alcohol and other factors on gastric ulcers, O. A. A. Bock has suggested that ulcers may be the product of an interaction between chronic stomach inflammation, acid and pepsin in the gastric juices, and one or more factors acting as a catalyst. He has concluded that acid by itself doesn't seem to be important in the production of gastric ulcers because, as we know, most patients with that kind of ulcer make normal or somewhat less than normal amounts of acid. It may be that acid represents nothing more than a key link in a chain of events preceding the development of ulcers and that some other catalytic factor such as alcohol then becomes essential.

In an often quoted study, O. Hagnell and G. Wretmark observed that in most cases of peptic ulcer in alcoholics that they had studied, the ulcer disorder had developed *before* alcohol abuse had begun. They concluded that the assumption that peptic ulcer was the secondary result of alcohol abuse was groundless. Alcoholics often use alcohol as a substitute for food, and perhaps it's not so much the alcohol as the poor diet that contributes to ulcers.

ASPIRIN

While the roles of coffee, tobacco and alcohol in the causation of ulcers are not entirely clear, aspirin *can* cause ulcers. Whether it's taken on an intermittent or a continuous basis, whether for headache, arthritis or other conditions, aspirin definitely damages the stomach lining. Aspirin may well be the most commonly self-prescribed medication. Many people aren't aware that this or that compound they're taking contains significant amounts of aspirin. In fact, for some of these medications, the aspirin may be the primary active ingredient, although the name and label may not actually reflect this.

Huge quantities of aspirin are consumed every year in the United States. The British are said to take 20 percent more aspirin than the Americans, while the Australians, perhaps the greatest consumers of aspirin in the world, take *two times* as much as the British. It's probably a tribute of some sort to the overall safety of the medication that we don't see more trouble from it than we do.

The first report suggesting that aspirin may damage the gastric lining appeared as early as 1938, but there's still considerable disagreement over the exact implications of this observation. From animal studies we know that a large amount of aspirin in the stomach irritates the gastric lining, but that this irritation decreases in intensity after a week or so despite continued administration of the drug. In humans, however, a number of factors may modify both the degree and the extent of the injury—the route by which the aspirin is taken (oral, rectal or intravenous), the amount consumed, the level of the acidity in the stomach at the time it's taken, and whether or not alcohol is taken at the same time. Even body tissue levels of vitamin C may affect the body's sensitivity to aspirin. Although it's possible to develop some tolerance for aspirin, making it somewhat less injurious even when taken continuously, irritation of the gastrointestinal tract causes an increased loss of blood in bowel movements. This blood loss, however small, continues as long as aspirin is taken on a regular basis.

Here is only a partial list of medications containing aspirin, many of which are simply sold over the counter in the United States, Britain and Australia.

COFFEE, TOBACCO, ALCOHOL AND ASPIRIN

COMMONLY USED PRODUCTS CONTAINING ASPIRIN

A.C.A.
A.P.C.
A.P.C. No. 2
A.P.C. pediatric
A.P.C. with
butalbital
A.P.C. with
codeine
A.S.A.
A.S.A. compound
Abactal
Ace-caf-edine
Acetabar
Aceticyl
Acetidine Nos. 1
and 2
Acetidine with
codeine
Acetol
Acetophen
Acetosal
Acetosalin
Acetphen-Acetyl
Acetycol
Acetylin
Acetylsalicylic
Acid
Acetysal
Aidant
Alasil
Alatal

Alka-Seltzer
Alka-Seltzer plus
cold medicine
Alprine
Ambrol
Aminat powder
Amphophen
Anacin
Anadin
Analdyne
Analexin
Analgia
Analgin
Andosix
Anexsia-D
Anexsia with
codeine
Angier's Junior
Aspirin
Ansemco Nos. 1,
2, and 5
Ansodyne
Antoin
Apac
Aphodyne
Aphophen
Ariphon
Arlcaps
Arthritis Strength
Bufferin
Asbarphen

Ascadin
As-ca-phen
Ascodeen-30
Ascriptin
Ascriptin A/D
Ascriptin with
codeine
Ascum
Askit powder,
tablets
Aspacam
Aspergum
Asphac-B
Asphac-G
Asphedex
Aspibarb
Aspidyne
Aspidyne com-
pound
Aspidyne with
codeine
Aspirdrops
Aspirfens
Aspirgran
Aspirin (all
brands)
Aspirin Dulcet
Aspirin-
Phenobarbital
Aspirin-
Secobarbital

SOURCES: C. N. Banks and J. H. Baron, "Drugs Containing Aspirin," *Lancet*, May 23, 1964, p. 1165. *Physicians' Desk Reference*, 31st ed. (1977), p. 303. "Take Your Medicine But Know What You're Taking First!" *Woman's Day*, March 8, 1977.

Aspirocal
Aspirjen
Aspiroffeine
Aspirotab
Aspirotab with
  codeine
Aspirpops
Aspivite
Aspodyne
Aspodyne with
  codeine
Aspriodine
Aspro
Asteric
Asteric compound
Axotal

Barbasprin
Bayer Aspirin
Bayer children's
  cold tablets
Bayer timed-
  release aspirin
Beecham's
  powder
Bellaspro with co-
  deine Nos. 1
  and 2
Beltona
Bemaco
Broprins
Bromo-Seltzer
Buff-A Comp
Buffadyne
Buffadyne 25
Bufferin

Cafdis
Calcium-Diuretin

Calurin
Cama Inlay-Tabs
Caprin
Capriton
Carrtone
Ce-K-Sal
Cephacan
Cephos
Chloro-Yeast
Cholisate
Cinbisal
Cirin
Clarke's Blood
  Mixture, tab-
  lets
Codadyne
Codasa
Codasphen
Codaspro Nos. 1
  and 2
Codeine com-
  pound
Codempiral
Codempiral Nos.
  2 and 3
Codesal
Codesal Nos. 1
  and 2
Codessin
Codilax
Codis
Codsal Nos. 1 and
  2
Cogesic 16
Colascorb
Colchipirine
Colchi-Sal
Colrex
Colrex compound

Colsalide
Congespirin
Conprin
Copavin com-
  pound
Cope
Cordex
Cordex-forte
Coricidin
Coricidin D
Coricidin Demi-
  lets for Children
Coricidin Medi-
  lets for Children
Cortadyne
Cortisal
Corydrane
Crystar
Cupal capsules
Cyclopal and
  aspirin
Cystex

Daisy powders,
  tablets
Dalca
Darvon Com-
  pound
Darvon Com-
  pound-65
Darvon with
  A.S.A.
Darvon-N with
  A.S.A.
Daprisal
Decagesic
Delenar
Dellipsoids D.4,
  D.5, and D.10

Dexocodeine
Disprin
Diuronil
Do-Do
Dolene Compound-65
Doloral
Doloxene Co.
Doluiran F.B.A.
Dorodol
Dristan
Drowz
Duradyne DHG Tablets
Duragesic

Ecotrin
Edrisal
Ekammon
Elestol
Empiral
Empirin
Empirin Compound
Empirin Compound with codeine phosphate Nos. 1, 2, 3, and 4
Emprazil
Emprazil-C
Encynex
Endo
Entrosalyl
Entrosalyl (Vitaminized)
Epragen
Equagesic
Equaprin

Excedrin
Excedrin P.M.
Exodyne
Exogen

Fennings Rheumatic Tablets
Fiorinal
Fiorinal with codeine
Florinal
For-Dyne
Formasal
Fuller Brand Celery Perles

Gelsodyne
Genasprin
Glutalate
Glutalate with prednisone
Gynopax

Harvadal
Hasacode
Hasamal
Henasphen
Hycetin
Hydrodyne
Hypnosed
Hypon

Ideopirine
Intrasept
Ioxantin
Ipral-Aspirin
Iromin

Junior Paynocil

Kaladex
Kalmopyrin
Kalsetal
Kandu
Kaputine
Kengesin
Kephaldol
Kestoma
Koray

Lumalgin
Lumaspirin with Hyoscyamus

Macprin
Measurin
Meclotin B.D.H.
Medadent
Medro-Cordex
Mensinole
Mepho-Dex
Methyl Aspriodine
Minac
Mincolate
Momentum

Natridiol
Nembudeine
Nembu-Gesic
Nembutal and aspirin
Neocylate
Neocylate HC
Neocylate (sodium-free)
Neocylate with codeine
Neocylate with colchicine

Neocylate with
cortisone
Neocylone
Neo-Saliciphen
Neurodyne
Nipirin
Norgesic
Nurse Sykes
powders
Nu-Seals aspirin
Nu-Seals sodium
salicylate

P.A.C. compound
Paadon
Pabalate HC
Pabalate (sodium-
free)
Pabirin Buffered
Tablets
Painex
Palaprin
Panalgesic
Paxedin
Paynocil
P-B-Sal-C
P-B-Sal-C
(sodium-free)
P-B-Sal-C (with
colchicine)
Pembrin
Pen-Phetamine
Peralga
Percodan
Percodan-Demi
Persistin
Phac
Phalcin

Phen-Acetyl
Phenaphen
Phenaphen Plus
Phensal
Phensic
Phoscodin
Pipergan
Pirisol
Pirseal
Pixylators
Plaquenil with
aspirin
Plus-Prin
Polygesic
Progesic Com-
pound-65
Propax
Propoxyphene
compound

Rasprin
Readers powders,
tablets
Regaspirin
Renipas powder
Rexall
Rheumaprin
Rhinex
Robaxisal
Ronazine
Ropad
Rumarid

S.A.C.
S.N.A.
Salcorbine
Salcort
Salcort-Delta

Saletin
Salibar JR
Salicitum
Salicol
Saliphen
Sali-Zem No. 2
Sal-So-Col
Salsprin
Sedax
Semapirin
Shadspro
Sigmagen
Sinco
Sine-Aid
Sine-Off
SK-65 Compound
Capsules
Solprin
Spira-Dine
Stero-Darvon
with A.S.A.
Stronicaps
Stuart Prolar
Stuart Prolar-B
Supac
Synalgos Capsules
Synalgos-D.C.
Capsules
Synirin

Tabaran
Tac-55
Tempogen
Tempogen Forte
Tercin
Tetride
Theryl
Topsy

Triaminicin	Uriliac	Viodox
Tycalsin		Vitanium
	Vagadil	Vitasprin
Ucal Children's	Vanquish	
soluble aspirin	Veganin	Wright's Capsules
Uniprin	Velox	Zactirin

Aspirin's effect on the gastric mucosa may be local, not generalized. Direct contact with the aspirin, rather than a more generalized response to the drug, may produce the injury. In one interesting study, patients about to undergo stomach surgery for ulcer were given aspirin the night before. During the operation, it was noted that the gastric mucosa had very localized areas of inflammation and even superficial ulcers, some of which conformed exactly to the fragments of aspirin tablet still lying in them.

In a recent article in the medical journal *Gut*, an Australian physician, Dr. J. M. Duggan, described a curious phenomenon to which attention had first been drawn by a series of papers published by B. P. Billington, also an Australian. During the early 1940's so many young women in eastern Australia developed gastric ulcers that it was a veritable "epidemic." Since the ulcers developed in young people living in a restricted geographic area, the observers concluded that an unidentified environmental factor was at fault. So many cases were involved that patterns of hospital admission for ulcer were changed. The ratio of male to female sufferers that had been established over a thirty-year period was reversed, females beginning to outnumber males.

According to a related study done by Duggan and B. L. Chapman, of sixty-one females with gastric ulcer, fifty-two, or over 85 percent, took at least two doses of aspirin preparation each week, most at least two a day. Four-fifths of these women took the aspirin in the form of an aspirin, phenacetin and caffeine compound sold over the counter.

Regular takers of aspirin tend to be predominantly middle-aged women, and a highly significant relationship exists between taking aspirin regularly for "chronic headache" or joint pains and the development of gastric ulcer. In one study, over 65 percent of seventy-seven hospital patients with a diagnosis of gastric ulcer consumed an average of four aspirin a day—three to seven times the average in that particular community. These patients were mostly younger middle-aged women. At the Mayo Clinic, it was found that more than 50 percent of gastric ulcer patients regularly took fifteen or more aspirin preparations each week. Only about one in ten patients in a control group of people without ulcers took that much. Men seem less inclined to be affected by aspirin than women are, but a significantly greater number of women take it.

A number of reports on the relationship between aspirin and ulcer note that patients tend to deny, for one reason or another, that they are taking the drug. Poor reporting naturally makes the data especially difficult to interpret. The denial may be based on a peculiar sense of embarrassment; or it may be a result of the fact that many patients simply don't know that the drugs they are taking contain aspirin.

I have noticed that a dismaying number of people with ulcers take compounds containing aspirin in an effort to *relieve the pain associated with ulcer*. Again, this seems to be related to the fact that they are not aware that the drug they are taking contains significant amounts of aspirin. Take, for example, the case of Lillian:

MELBOURNE, AUSTRALIA. 2:10 P.M., JULY 14, 1971

Lillian is a forty-seven-year-old housewife who's sitting in her family doctor's office waiting to be seen. Although she complains of chronic mild headaches and occasional stiffness in her fingers and shoulders, her main trouble is a bellyache of three months' duration. Elaborate examination reveals nothing seriously wrong with her, but x-rays of her stomach show an active gastric ulcer.

Under careful and persistent questioning, she denies taking any drugs or medications. Not a smoker or a drinker, she has only two to three cups of tea a day. She has no family history of ulcers, is happily married and doesn't feel especially stressed by her life.

After two months of therapy characterized by a bland diet, antacids and tranquilizers, she complains to her physician that the medicines he prescribed haven't helped and that even the Bufferin she takes, some eight to twelve tablets a day, make her stomach hurt. When asked why she didn't tell the doctor she takes aspirin, she denies she does. "It's Bufferin, not aspirin," she says, "and besides, it's not a drug —everyone takes it, don't they?"

There is, then, almost certainly an association between erosions of the gastric lining, bleeding from the stomach, and taking aspirin. Prolonged aspirin use can lead to the development of chronic *gastric* ulcer. The effect of the use of aspirin on *duodenal* ulcer is not as clear, but there's less likely to be a relationship here.

The precise way in which aspirin causes ulcer isn't entirely apparent, but it may be due to a direct toxic effect by the medication rather than to a generalized systemic one. The combination of aspirin and alcohol is particularly devastating. *No one with known ulcer should take aspirin or aspirin-containing compounds in any form.* Alternative pain relievers are available and should be used instead.

7

Racial, Geographic, Nutritional, Political and Social Factors

It can be said that each civilization has a pattern of disease peculiar to it. The pattern of disease is an expression of the response of man to his total environment (physical, biological, and social); the response is, therefore, determined by anything that affects man himself or his environment.
                                    —René J. Dubos (1901–   )

Darwinian fitness is compounded of a mutual relationship between the organism and the environment . . . in fundamental characteristics the actual environment is the fittest possible abode of life.
                        —Lawrence J. Henderson (1878–1942),
                        The Fitness of the Environment

In looking for a place to retire, the great playwright George Bernard Shaw supposedly visited graveyards in hamlets throughout the Irish and English countryside, scrutinizing headstones to determine the longevity of different areas' inhabitants. Apparently he chose well—he lived to the ripe old age of ninety-four!

An astute observer of the human condition, Shaw apparently believed that geographic factors were a key to long life. He recognized that some intangible, perhaps the air or the water or something in the soil, contributed to a healthier environment. While somewhat naive, as it does not take internal factors into account, his notion may help explain why certain people get ulcers and others do not. Geographic, climatic, geopolitical, and sociocultural factors undoubtedly have subtly affected who gets ulcers and why.

But as with many other aspects of the problem, it's easy to oversimplify. Due to all sorts of emotional and physical factors, people tend to react in very individual ways to virtually identical environmental pressures. What seems unbearably stressful to some people may not even be noticed by others. There's an old anecdote about a man who visits his doctor with complaints of a bellyache. The doctor examines him and then tells him he has an ulcer. "It must be my job," the man says. He tells the doctor that he sorts oranges by size all day. When the doctor points out that this kind of work doesn't seem very stressful, the man replies, "But, Doc, it's the *decisions* that're driving me nuts!"

The constantly changing ratio of male to female ulcer sufferers, the fluctuating frequency of duodenal as compared to gastric ulcers, and the shifting geographic distribution of ulcers are all testimony to the fact that the disorder is dynamic. As long as scientists have collected statistics on people with ulcers, there've been innumerable qualitative and quantitative shifts in who gets them, where and why.

We know, for example, that gastric ulcers used to be as common or more common than duodenal ulcers. They no longer are. We also know that stomach ulcers were more common in young women around the turn of the century than in young women today.* Take the story of Melissa.

LONDON, ENGLAND. 6:05 P.M., DECEMBER 24, 1897

A twenty-seven-year-old mother of two, Melissa is dressing for a Christmas Eve banquet at her father-in-law's home. She is a pretty, well-groomed Victorian lady, always elegantly coiffured and attired. Her figure is a classic of the times, which she manages to keep shapely by compressing her normally twenty-four-inch waist into a svelte eighteen inches by tightly lacing her corset. She's wealthy and happily married; in fact, her only complaint is frequent abdominal "soreness" after eating.

Her dressing completed, Melissa is radiant and right-up-to-the-minute fashionable. Melissa has a gastric ulcer.

An "epidemic" of peptic ulcers that began in the 1920's probably reached its peak in the late fifties and early sixties, then diminished, and now shows evidence of increasing again. All of these observations contribute to our understanding of the disorder, and may have some value in predicting the future.

Almost all attempts to identify specific occupational, environmental and sociological factors as a cause for ulcers have been frustrated by problems inherent in the methods available for gathering data. Often, studies done using the currently available approaches yield contradictory findings, sometimes because each investigator is measuring something different and sometimes because the very instrument of measurement is inadequate or mishandled.

---

* Some have attributed the high frequency of ulcers in young women of the Victorian era to the clothes then fashionable—specifically, to pressure on the stomach from the tight lacing of corsets. In fact, some have suggested that the switch from braces (suspenders) to belts may have increased the incidence of gastric ulcers seen today in men.

If, for example, one wishes to study the prevalence of ulcers, it would seem logical to refer to hospital records. But as M. Susser, a British epidemiologist, has pointed out, different groups have different access to medical care: for instance, Philadelphians are far more likely to be hospitalized for ulcers than are African Bantus; military personnel have better access to medical care than do migratory agricultural workers; and so forth.

Sometimes when they are questioned people who have definitely been hospitalized for ulcers either forget or actually deny the episode. In one study 20 percent neglected to report it. Sometimes sociocultural factors affect the number of hospital admissions. In parts of the Orient or Africa, where the hospitalization of a patient often implies his impending death or is construed as a family affair in which relatives join him in the hospital, people are often unwilling to go to the hospital. Finally, the availability of skilled physicians and sophisticated diagnostic techniques may significantly increase the quality of information obtainable from hospital records.

Susser questions whether a study of mortality figures would be of help in determining the incidence of ulcers. From simple death rates in a community, or even from autopsy studies, one might conclude that ulcers are far less common than they actually are. In comparison to heart disease, stroke and cancer, ulcer kills relatively few people each year. But while it may not be a leading cause of death, it is a very common disorder.

Another possible source of help in determining the incidence of ulcers is a study of the frequency of complications that normally require medical attention and hospitalization. The perforated peptic ulcer, the massively bleeding ulcer, and the ulcer-causing obstruction of the outlet to the stomach are not very likely to go unreported by the patient. However, not all ulcers bleed, not all ulcers perforate, and not all ulcers obstruct. Also, complications are more frequent in gastric than in duodenal ulcers; older patients tend to have more complications than younger ones; men tend to have more complications than women.

Despite these limitations, we do the best with what we have. Susser concluded a particularly articulate analysis of the problems by stating that "the difficulties of epidemiologic studies in peptic ulcer are not so formidable as to preclude their use. They have in fact contributed a great deal and much more can be learned from them."

RACIAL FACTORS

Race is one of the factors that has been considered in the search to identify groups of people who are especially prone to the development of ulcers. While nothing conclusive has been found, some interesting observations have been made. People with blood group type O have a higher than normal risk of ulcers. Since the distribution of blood type O varies slightly from race to race, this area of investigation has been pursued with some vigor. But since it's next to impossible to distinguish racial factors from social, geographic and cultural ones, careful interpretation of the reported "facts" is essential.

For example, while cases of peptic ulcers are relatively infrequent in blacks, particularly in Africa, recent studies suggest that the disease is not as uncommon as was once thought. According to some studies, ulcers are very rare among Kenyan blacks and South African Bantus, but according to others done among blacks from Uganda and Zanzibar, cases of ulcers are not all that infrequent. These are examples of variability in the correlation of race with ulcers (race plus geography). In some studies gastric ulcers were found to be about twice as common in white as in black males, while the incidence among females seems to be relatively constant. A multiplicity of factors (race plus sex) may also be at play here.

Other information casts doubt on the importance of race in the development of ulcers. Among Nordic peoples, for example, the death rate for males with ulcers is low for Finns and very high for Norwegians. The death rate for duodenal ulcer is very low for Swedish men but high for Danes and Norwegians. These observations hold true even if the people studied aren't living in their homeland, and they are based on investigations carried out in more than twenty different nations.

These observations lead to the conclusion that racial factors aren't nearly so critical in the development of ulcers as was once thought. Despite the distortions that may result from the relatively crude techniques we use to study such influences, other factors have to be considered.

GEOGRAPHIC FACTORS

Does where you live make a difference in susceptibility? There are enormous differences in the frequency of people with ulcers, not only in countries throughout the world, but in different regions of the same country.

For example, in Java, a high rate of ulcer is found among Chinese coolies but a low rate among Indians. That race alone is not a factor here can be seen by the low incidence of ulcers in Chinese living on the mainland. The frequency of ulcers in southern Nigeria differs markedly from that in northern Nigeria, and the frequency in southern India from that in northern India. Even complications from ulcers vary on a geographic basis: for example, acute perforations of ulcer are seen twice as often in Aberdeen, Scotland, as in York, England, only a short distance away.

Townspeople consistently have more ulcers than people who live in rural areas. It would be easy to misinterpret this as a reflection of the faster pace of life in the cities, but although *men* in cities definitely have a higher incidence of ulcers, the frequency of ulcers in women who live in towns is not significantly different from that of those who live on the farm.

You can readily see that it's almost impossible to say that this or that specific geographic element causes ulcers. The marked variation in ulcer incidence from country to country, from racial group to racial group within the same country, and within the same racial group dispersed among different countries means that geographic differences *alone* can't account for these widely divergent observations.

NUTRITIONAL INFLUENCES

Many people consider diet to be extremely important in the development of ulcers. Although techniques for collecting such data are as cumbersome as those used in the study of racial and geographic factors and are notably unreliable, some statistics support this assumption. For example, prior to 1918 the ulcer rate in Russia was very low—about one or two sufferers for every two hundred people. Following the great famine in this country after the Revolution and World War I, the incidence rose approximately *fifteen-fold.* As the political situation stabilized, food became more plentiful and the frequency of ulcers is said to have decreased again to pre-1918 levels. Was this due to diet or to politics? Or to both?

A fairly large body of evidence gathered from animal experiments leads to the conclusion that some nutritional deficiencies can cause gastric ulcers. Diets deficient in protein and vitamins A, B, and C have resulted in stomach damage ranging from minor, relatively superficial erosions to actual through-and-through perforation in dogs, guinea pigs, rats, chicks and monkeys.*

There is *some* human evidence, too. People living in certain parts of India and Ethiopia, where people's diets are notably deficient in protein and in vitamins A and B, have a relatively high rate of ulcers. The difference in ulcer rate between the natives of northern India, where ulcers are practically unknown, and those of southern India, where the ulcer rate is high, may be based in part on the different eating habits of the two groups.

However, several studies on the effect of malnutrition in causing or reactivating ulcers suggest that certain dietary deficiencies may actually prevent them. In black South Africa, for example, there is a low incidence of ulcer and a high rate of liver disease due to deficient diets. Since the liver plays an important role in the metabolism and elimination of female sex hormones (which are also produced to a certain extent in the male), these hormones may rise to abnormal levels in men, causing atrophy of the testicles and enlarged breasts. This change in hormonal milieu in the South Africans may protect them from ulcers, since research shows that high estrogen levels may account for the markedly lower incidence of ulcers in women as compared to men.

Also, the little evidence we have from studies of concentration camp victims in World War II doesn't support the notion that malnutrition is an important cause of ulcers.

---

* A major problem with these investigations is that the animals' stomachs may not be truly analogous to human stomachs. In addition to anatomic and physiologic differences between animals and humans, spontaneous ulcer development in lower animals is uncommon except in a rare species and under unusual circumstances. So while much valuable information has been obtained from dogs, rats, chicks, monkeys, pigs and other species, it's difficult to apply the data gained from animal studies to humans.

They were rare in such inmates despite widespread starvation, and occurred in significant numbers only after these people were freed.

Thus the data derived from studies done on the relationship between diet and ulcers is both confusing and contradictory. With the exceptions of protein and some vitamins, it's difficult to identify specific nutritional factors that may cause ulcers in people.

SEASONAL AND CLIMATIC FACTORS

Many investigators have examined the possibility of a relationship between certain seasonal and climatic factors and the development of ulcers. The rationale for such investigations is fairly simple. Epidemiologic studies have demonstrated that everywhere in the world hospital admissions for such disorders as coronary artery disease, schizophrenia and other mental diseases—not to mention suicide—vary on a monthly basis, and have identifiable seasonal peaks. As Hippocrates himself once said: "Whoever wishes to pursue properly the science of medicine must proceed thus: first he ought to consider what effect each season of the year can produce; for the seasons are not alike, but differ widely both in themselves and at their changes. For with the season men's diseases, like their digestive organs, suffer change."

Could Hippocrates, several millennia ago and with nothing more than intuition and primitive observation, have stumbled on a truth? In both humans and animals the volume and the acidity of gastric juices and the incidence and severity of dyspeptic symptoms, as well as the complications of ulcers, seem to be greater in the autumn and in the spring than during other periods of the year. This holds true in at least some of the countries studied, including the United States. Surveys done in various parts of the world have shown a peak incidence in the onset of new ulcers or flare-up of existing ulcer in every month except July. Near the equator, however, where there is a constant mild climate year-round (such as, for example, in parts of Mexico or Brazil), there seems to be no seasonal variation in incidence. Perhaps constancy of climate and moderate temperatures flatten out the seasonal cycles. But then how do we explain the fact that a month-to-month study done in Switzerland, with its marked variations in seasonal climate, reveals no change at all?

In northern Norway the peak period for ulcer recurrence, or the discovery of new cases, runs from January through April, but in western Norway it's from November through January. In Australia the peak seems to occur in May and June. Perforated ulcers occur most frequently in December in London and west Scotland, but in northeast Scotland they occur more frequently during the summertime.

Studies have even been done on the correlations between ulcer flare-ups and the time of day or the day of the week. In Scotland, for example, perforated ulcers occur more frequently toward the end of the morning and the end of the afternoon; they are most frequent on Friday and Saturday, and are relatively uncommon on Sunday and Monday. Unsuccessful attempts have also been made to correlate flare-ups of ulcer symptoms with environmental temperature, barometric pressure and humidity.

High altitude has been incriminated as a contributory factor in the development of ulcers—probably with some validity. An extraordinarily high number of Peruvian miners, who work at very high altitudes, suffer from gastric ulcer. In an article in *Gastroenterology* G. Klinge and L. Peña reported that among these natives stomach ulcers are twenty times more common than duodenal ulcer, a remarkable reversal of the normal ratio. Moreover, these people get stomach ulcers at a very early age (most are males in their twenties), and almost all of them hemorrhage and require surgery—most on an emergency basis.

Various unusual elements of the life style of these miners

make it difficult to incriminate any single factor as a cause for their type of ulcer disorder. Their diets are low in protein and vitamins; what food they have is poor in quality; they are heavy drinkers and cocaine users. Furthermore, their blood is much thicker and richer than the blood of people who live at or near sea level, an attempt on the part of their bodies to compensate for the thinness of the air they breathe.

This abnormal increase in the number of red cells circulating in the blood (polycythemia) and in the volume of blood (hypervolemia) tends to slow the circulation and increases the tendency for blood clots to form in small vessels. Since gastric ulcers are also seen in people who suffer from polycythemia vera, an abnormal blood condition similarly characterized by polycythemia and hypervolemia, it's appealing to conclude that these factors may play a role in causing the Peruvian miners' ulcers. The small blood vessels of the gastric lining may clot, depriving it of oxygen and nutrients and making it more susceptible to destruction. In any event, the effects of high altitude and the characteristic life style of these miners on the frequency of ulcers—particularly in the stomach rather than in the duodenum—seem real. These observations are also further evidence that gastric ulcers and duodenal ulcers are two different diseases.

Again, however, no pat conclusions can be drawn. Studies carried out in Canada, a country with widely variable seasonal extremes, showed that ulcer incidence is *not* related to extreme temperature, barometric pressure, total radiation from the sun and sky, total rain- or snowfall, or wind force and direction.

WAR AND STRESS

If stress has a role in causing ulcer, periods of widespread economic or political upheaval should bring with them change in both the incidence and the severity of ulcers. In fact, this seems to be the case. The aforementioned startling fifteen-fold increase in ulcers noted in Russia during the 1918 chaos brought on by the Revolution and World War I supports this notion. World War II also offered some unusual opportunities to study these phenomena at close hand.

LONDON, ENGLAND. 9:42 P.M., MAY 26, 1940

Darrold is a sixty-nine-year-old white man, a former tram driver. He's hiding in the cellar of his modest flat, crouched under a heavy table surrounded by sandbags. For the last twenty minutes he has been listening to the incessant percussive pounding of exploding German bombs. It is another night of the blitz.

Darrold's greatest fear is not for himself, but for his widowed daughter and grandchild, who share his protected cubbyhole. He has had intermittent "indigestion" for almost four months, although he's been otherwise healthy all his life.

He feels a sudden searing pain in his abdomen and for a moment thinks that he has been hit by a piece of flying glass. He says nothing, checking only to see that everyone else is all right. Sixteen minutes later the "all clear" sounds. He's near collapse, but his daughter manages to get him to a nearby hospital. Because of the number of injured bombing victims, he receives no medical attention for five hours. When he's finally examined, no wounds are found on his abdomen. A sharp-witted physician, however, makes the diagnosis of a perforated peptic ulcer. Within three more hours he is operated upon, but due to complications he will die sixteen days later.

In another part of the city a similar tale unfolds.

John, a twenty-seven-year-old white male who at ten lost his left leg in a cycling accident, has been working as an ambulance helper. He's trapped in a shelter during the raid. Although he has had no previous symptoms of any kind, he too experiences a sudden very severe abdominal pain. He makes his own way to the hospital and within hours is operated upon for perforated ulcer. *He* will do well, however, and leave the hospital in eight days.

Both of these men are "bloodless" victims of the blitz.

An increased frequency in the development of ulcers occurred during wartime in Denmark, Holland, Sweden, Germany, Switzerland, the United States, Belgium and Austria. In Germany the incidence of new ulcer almost doubled annually between 1938 and 1940 when compared to 1937 to 1938. Duodenal ulcer roughly doubled in frequency, while gastric ulcer quadrupled. In Switzerland an over 30 percent increase in ulcers occurred during 1940 to 1942, when compared to the 1937–1939 period. During the same era the frequency of perforations of gastric ulcer rose almost 35 percent, and that of bleeding from gastric ulcer almost 25 percent.

M. Kretchmer and N. Markoff both studied the increased ulcer frequency in Switzerland. Each found that the rise was due not only to recurrences in old cases but also to the development of new ones. Kretchmer attributed the increase to nervous tension and fear of German invasion, while Markoff thought it was due to a diet relatively low in protein and high in vegetable roughage.

The observations made in England during the blitz are especially convincing. Hospital records for the period from 1929 to 1940 show a relatively stable rate of admissions for treatment of ulcers. Then in the fall of 1940, the point at which the really heavy raiding on London began, deaths from all kinds of peptic ulcer increased in both men and women.

Shortly after the beginning of the second week in September 1940, seven patients with perforated peptic ulcers were admitted within a few days of one another to the Charing Cross Hospital in London, which normally admitted only one such patient a month. In a unique evaluation of the phenomenon based on information from sixteen different London hospitals, D. N. Stewart and D. M. Winser were able to show a statistically significant increase in perforated peptic ulcers during the first two months of heavy air raids (September and October 1940). They concluded that the probable cause for the increase was anxiety.

I'm relatively comfortable with these data, but a few caveats must be entered. The fact that the statistics used to determine frequency of ulcers are drawn from hospital records alone prevents these studies from being "perfect." A huge slice of the population (healthy young men) may well have been out of the country at the time. Those remaining behind would certainly have been older and composed of a greater percentage of relatively infirm people. Men with known ulcers might have been excluded from military service and kept behind performing other duties.

Still another fly in the ointment comes from two separate studies from Germany.

STALINGRAD, RUSSIA. JANUARY 3, 1943

Heinz is a twenty-nine-year-old front-line infantryman who's been in active combat since Hitler attacked Russia on June 22, 1941. In civilian life Heinz was an unskilled worker at the Daimler-Benz Automotive Works in Stuttgart, Germany. A shy, quiet and somewhat retiring person, at twenty-four he developed a duodenal ulcer, which—although it flared up only intermittently—was nevertheless bothersome right up until the time he was inducted into the army. (Elsewhere the ulcer might well have kept him out of the service.)

Heinz has been in the thick of the ferocious counteroffensives launched by the Russians in November 1942. He's tired, frequently hungry, cold, wet and almost perpetually frightened. Still, quite remarkably, he hasn't had a flare-up of his ulcer since the day he entered the army. There's been no abdominal pain for almost two years.

Heinz's story could easily be dismissed if his was an isolated case. But this notion is refuted by a study of more than fifty war veterans known to have had peptic ulcers before their induction into the service. These men were notably free of complaints while in service at the front. If fear and anxiety is a crucial factor in causing ulcers, how do we explain the experiences of these soldiers? Moreover, how do we explain the fact that after the men were discharged from the service, their ulcers tended to flare up again?

These two contradictory sets of evidence seem to me to emphasize again that one's response to the environment is extremely personal and individual. What was threatening to Heinz in his civilian life may not have been present at all during his life in the service. People often feel more comfortable in a highly regimented institution or occupation than in an open-ended situation. We are all familiar with stories about men who after years of imprisonment simply can't make it in the outside world. As a matter of fact, the little information available concerning life in the World War II concentration camps leads one to believe that the frequency of ulcers in inmates was low—until they were freed, at which point it rose. M. Pflanz and his coworkers also noted that exclusion or forced expulsion from a community or group coincided with astonishing frequency with the onset or relapse of the peptic ulcer.

The search for a clue—any clue—as to a possible causative factor in the development of ulcers has been intense and widespread. We researchers have all been guilty of an almost desperate desire to find a common denominator in the various population groups known to have a high incidence (or a low incidence) of ulcers. So far we've unearthed only a few highly suggestive but not wholly convincing factors—high altitude and thin air as a contributor to gastric ulcers in Peruvian miners; some nutritional factors in population groups deprived of protein and vitamins A and B; stress caused by the heavy bombing raids of the blitz. But these aren't frivolous searches. They are studies performed by responsible, interested and trained observers. It is simply a measure of the variability of the ulcer disorder that so few incriminating solid data have emerged.

8

Genes, the Family Environment and Ulcers

People make people, not just by breeding them but by shaping one another's behavior.

—Nigel Calder,
The Human Conspiracy

All happy families resemble each other, each unhappy family is unhappy in its own way.

—Leo Tolstoi,
Anna Karenina

Two hundred years of the Industrial Revolution have naturally brought more than a simple change from an agriculturally oriented society to an urbanized one. Complain if you will about the postal service, but the pony express never stood a chance against it! Advances in technology—telephone, television and air travel—have contributed to an upheaval in the patterns of our lives. New social values and mores have deeply affected us. A major casualty of these changes has been the extended family.

The old-style family structure of several generations living near one another—the basis of small-town and rural America—has given way to the urban nuclear family, a smaller unit typically made up of one or both parents and their offspring, often quite far removed from their place of birth and from the kinds of warmth, discipline and support that came from the extended family. Sociologists tell us that there are inherent weaknesses in the nuclear-family way of life. Evidence of this can be found in the soaring crime rates, the spiraling divorce rates, hordes of runaway and disenfranchised children, and a growing disrespect for long-established religious, academic, social and governmental institutions.

The twentieth century has brought with it two world wars, the dislocation of millions upon millions of people from their homelands, and an increased acceptance of—or at least a passive response to—public and private immorality, with no end in sight. This period of cataclysmic change happens to coincide with a very high prevalence of ulcers, but are they truly related?

Patterns of health and disease undoubtedly reflect people's responses to profound societal changes. The ulcer epidemic that began in the early part of this century may well reflect the upheavals resulting from industrialization and the mass migrations of the last two centuries. But the controversy as to whether heredity or environment predominates in causing ulcers is as yet unresolved. There is evidence supporting both sides.

The study of family environmental and hereditary factors may help us understand the complexity inherent in the question of heredity versus environment as a cause of ulcers. Woody's case is a good one to look at.

TOPEKA, KANSAS. 7:45 A.M., APRIL 16, 1976

Woodrow is a twenty-eight-year-old machinist about to undergo surgery for a bleeding duodenal ulcer. Woody knows quite a bit about ulcers. Not only has he suffered from one for more than twelve years, but his grandfather, his father, two of his five brothers, one of his two sisters, and a niece and nephew all have ulcers. Eight family members spanning four generations have been coping with the disorder for almost fifty years. The future for this family, at least in terms of ulcers, seems dim.

Ever since the family first settled in this country some five generations ago, its history has been somewhat checkered; it is not a stable group, with more than its share of multiple marriages and divorces, runaway children, serious brushes with the law, and lazy and mentally unstable members. It has fragmented and dispersed, no one city having more than three family members living in it. None of these people can really tell you where they are from. They only know where they are now.

Woody will survive his operation and emerge "cured." What the future holds for his family, however, one can only guess.

This case is an admittedly extreme example of peptic ulcers as a family affair. While not everyone with an ulcer has a relative who also has one, ulcers are two to three times more frequent in relatives of people with ulcers than one would expect, compared with the distribution of ulcers in the general population.

Also, people suffering from duodenal ulcer tend to have relatives with duodenal ulcers, and people with gastric ulcer tend to have parents or siblings afflicted with gastric ulcer. But is this a result of genetic inheritance (is it transmitted by the genes?) or of the family environment—that is to say, the interaction between members of a family group and their life style.

The role of hereditary factors in any disease process is rarely clear-cut. The acknowledged psychosomatic nature of ulcers simply makes the problem more difficult. As K. L. Becker points out, collecting accurate information on human "pedigrees" is very hard, and there are a number of ways serious errors can be made. Sometimes the number of off-spring are too few to analyze with any degree of accuracy. Long periods of time between generations, untraceable illegitimate offspring, and selective telling or out-and-out mis-representation of the facts commonly hamper the researcher's efforts to collect precise information. Distinguishing environmental from genetic factors is an almost hopeless task.

According to a Swedish study, ulcers were twice as common among the 319 living brothers of 102 male ulcer patients as in a control group, and both the fathers and the mothers of these ulcer patients had a significantly higher frequency of ulcers. Based on these data, as well as numerous other studies, the high occurrence of ulcers in certain families has been attributed not to common environmental factors but to a constitutional predisposition based on heredity.

The distribution of blood group types in various populations also provides support for the view that ulcers are genetically transmitted, because these distributions are slightly but significantly different from what one would expect based on normal population samples. The study of blood groups and their distribution in various populations is a time-honored technique for searching out genetic causes of disease. The blood type is easily determined and reliably predictable. Most important, it is *indisputably* genetically transmitted.

People with blood type O are about 35 percent more liable to develop duodenal ulcers than are people with blood group types A, B and AB. On the other hand, gastric ulcers are not as strongly associated with people with any particular blood group type, although type A is slightly more frequently seen.

Exactly why people with a certain blood type should be more prone to ulcers can't be fully explained. Some people have the ability to actually secrete the ABO blood type substances (antigens) in their saliva and other gastrointestinal juices. Since those of us who do *not* secrete these materials are about twice as liable to develop ulcers as those who do, it may be that their presence in our stomach's juices acts as a protective mechanism. Furthermore, people with blood type O who are also incapable of secreting the blood group antigens are about two and a half times more likely to develop an ulcer than are people with other blood types who do secrete them. Lastly, there seems to be an association between ulcer patients with blood type O and some of the complications of ulcers. Hemorrhaging and perforation of ulcers are more common in this group.

The role of heredity, however—at least when one looks only at the evidence available from studies of blood groups— is uncertain. Although Caucasians and Negroes with duodenal ulcers are *more* likely to have type O blood and *less* likely to have type A blood, this doesn't hold true for all races. In an obscure but interesting study of southwestern American Indians in Arizona, Nevada, California and Utah, M. L. Sievers and J. R. Marquis of the U.S. Public Health Service Indian hospital in Phoenix report that duodenal ulcers aren't often seen in these populations despite the fact that an average of 83 percent of these people have blood type O. Only 45 percent of Caucasians are type O. Inarguable evidence that ulcers are genetically transmittable, if such evidence exists at all, must be sought elsewhere.

Another way to seek out genetic determinants of diseases is to compare their frequency in different racial groups. We have long suspected that ulcer is more common among Caucasians than among blacks, although the difference isn't nearly so great as was once believed. Studies of blacks, Orientals and Caucasians have shown marked differences in the tendency to develop ulcers.

Still another way to study the relative importance of genetic and familial factors in the cause of illness is by analyzing information on twins. Although the common genetic background of identical twins is indisputable, the fact that twins grow up in a very similar environment—for example, having the same parents; living in the same home; attending the same schools and often the same classes; sharing remarkably similar dietary, sleep and work habits—makes for a fuzzy distinction between inherited and acquired traits.

Only a small body of literature exists on twins and ulcers, mainly because twins are comparatively rare. These studies are based on comparisons between identical and fraternal pairs of twins. If a specific disorder occurs more or less often in identical as opposed to fraternal twins, this could indicate that genetic factors are involved in the development of the given disease. Of course, as G. Eberhard, a pioneer in the field, has pointed out, these methods are based on the assumption that the environment—the world around us—affects identical and fraternal twins in the same way, particularly with regard to the trait being studied.

Twin studies have produced only inconclusive results. Eberhard did find that an increased sensitivity to stress combined with an "impaired" defense mechanism appeared to be the main trait of the ulcer twins he studied. He stated that "if an individual with low tolerance to distress and insufficient defense mechanisms is subjected to an emotional strain of a kind such that his self-esteem is threatened, a nervous-hormonal discharge is possible." This view is consistent with what we already know about the physiologic cause of ulcers.

His studies provided no evidence of any "typical" peptic ulcer personality. He supported Alexander's concept that a psychic conflict may precipitate the development of an ulcer, but he concluded that the factors of greatest importance for the etiology of ulcers are hereditary.

The following example of a pair of identical twins shows some of the problems inherent in studies of this type.

BIRMINGHAM, ALABAMA. MARCH 24, 1977

Sylvia and Sarah are fifty-seven-year-old identical twins. Sylvia has a gastric ulcer, but Sarah doesn't and has never had any abdominal complaints.

Both women were married by the time they were twenty-five, and initially both were happy, producing two children each. Sylvia first developed her ulcer at thirty-seven, during a period in which she was going through a divorce. Since that time she's had frequent flare-ups followed by periods of no symptoms. She's been hospitalized three times in the last five years, twice for hemorrhage requiring blood transfusions. Surgery was suggested, but she refused. She continued to have symptoms, but up until the present time no further complications have appeared.

The twins' mother was also known to have gastric ulcer, although their grandparents, their father and three other siblings besides Sarah are free of the disorder. The twins grew up in a small town outside of Birmingham, where their father managed a gas station and garage. He was a rather severe disciplinarian, harsh and restrictive, in contrast to their mother, who was mild-mannered, good-natured and warm. Nevertheless, it was felt to be a happy household, and the twins always got along well with each other as well as with their siblings. There was no rivalry between them, and neither independent observers nor the twins themselves considered either as dominant.

Both twins are extremely sensitive to criticism and describe themselves as anxious, tense, moody and sometimes "overenthusiastic." Both are characterized as short-tempered with a tendency to be quarrelsome and irritable. Sylvia is considerably more uptight than Sarah, who is warmer and more approachable. Sarah is more independent than Sylvia.

In this case both the genetic and the environmental factors appear to be remarkably similar; the twins even have similar personalities. Despite their apparently similar response to their environment, one developed ulcers in reaction to a major stress (marital discord and divorce), while the other, who never experienced such an emotional trauma, did not.

These observations suggest that the genetic factors in causing ulcer are possible, but weak. We can speculate that if Sylvia's marital life had been more tranquil she might not have developed an ulcer. Alternatively, if Sarah's marital situation had ended traumatically or if she'd experienced another kind of special crisis, she too might have developed an ulcer.

An excellent study carried out in Denmark on almost 600 pairs of twins (144 of the pairs were identical twins, and 209 of the pairs were fraternal twins of the same sex), in which at least one member of each pair had an ulcer, provides us with more evidence on this topic. Both members of the identical twin pairs had a significantly higher percentage of ulcers than did both members of the fraternal ones. Also, the fraternal twins of the same sex had a significantly higher rate of ulcer in both members of the pair than did the fraternal twins of opposite sex. The researchers, B. Harvald and M. Hauge, concluded that the familial concentration of ulcer cases is almost certainly due to shared environmental factors and not to shared genes.

Since all diseases are to some extent genetic in origin and to some extent environmental, we can safely conclude that the same holds true for ulcers. The evidence available seems to suggest that while genetic factors clearly are involved, environmental factors and the individual's interpretation of them are more important.

9

Ulcers in Women

Because of their vices, women . . . have put off their womanly nature and are therefore condemned to suffer the diseases of men.

—Seneca (4?B.C.–A.D. 65),
Moral Epistles to Lucilus

No one who is not female can be in a position to make accurate statements about women.

—Otto Weininger (1800–1903),
Sex and Character

Ever since just before the turn of the nineteenth century, the roles of both men and women in Western society have been changing at a dizzying rate. In contrast to their traditional role as wife, housekeeper and child-rearer, women today constitute almost half the work force in the United States; about a third of mothers with children under six are wage earners. Indeed, more and more women want to work each year, some for economic reasons but many in order to establish an identity of their own, apart from that of their husband.

As a psychosomatic disorder, ulcers are a prime example of the kind of health problem one would expect to reflect this cultural revolution. We do know that ulcer in women is a disorder that has undergone radical alterations in character over the last eighty or ninety years. Today peptic and especially duodenal ulcer is predominantly a male disorder, whereas before the turn of the century ulcers were roughly equally distributed between men and women. Before that, women seemed to predominate. Although poor record-keeping and the fact that duodenal and gastric ulcer were often lumped together may make generalizations about earlier periods suspect, studies from Britain and the United States seem to corroborate them.

The shift to ulcers being a predominantly male disorder began about ten years earlier in America than in England. By World War I there were six men with ulcers for every woman, and by the years of the Great Depression twelve to sixteen men suffered from the ailment for every woman who had it.

We also know that while the difference between the number of males with ulcers and the number of female ulcer sufferers is present even in infants and children, it doesn't really become meaningful until the children grow past puberty. During adolescence and thereafter the gap widens sharply. Whereas in prepubescent children the ratio of male to female ulcer sufferers varies from nearly equal to about 3.5 males to every female, the discrepancy increases and reaches peak proportions in the thirty-to-forty age group.

We can only guess why men are more vulnerable to the development of ulcer than women. An easy but somewhat shallow answer could be that modern society imposes greater stress on men than on women. Or that women have traditionally been permitted to express their emotions more openly and in a more socially acceptable way, while men are encouraged to repress their emotions.

GEOGRAPHIC AND RACIAL FACTORS

All over the world, wherever ulcer has been studied, it has been observed that men develop the disorder far more frequently than women. But when the overall incidence of ulcer varies from time to time within a country, or from one country to another, it's usually the male rate that changes. The female rate tends to remain relatively constant.

It's well established that the frequency of ulcer is higher in urban than in rural areas. But rural and urban women appear to get ulcers at about the same rate—it's the frequency of ulcers in men that accounts for the rural/urban difference. There's evidence that blacks are less vulnerable than whites. Here too, the discrepancy lies in the incidence of ulcers in males, not in females.

The question of whether the new status of women in modern society is affecting the rate at which they develop ulcers is an important one. But reliable information on this is not available. The ulcer rate seems to have dropped for both sexes; but, as best as can be determined, the male rate fell faster than the female rate.

If we think of ulcers as resulting from a constellation of forces—genetic, familial, occupational, dietary and so forth—a change in one or more of them can account for an *overall* drop in frequency of ulcers in both men and women. If, then, the male rate fell faster than the female rate, a *relative* net increase in the number of women with ulcers might occur. This in fact seems to be the case.

HORMONAL FACTORS AND ULCERS IN WOMEN

Ulcers in women are different from ulcers in men. Ulcer incidence in males only really gains momentum after boys reach sexual maturity. Pregnancy retards the development and activity of ulcers. The rate of development of a new ulcer or aggravation of an already existing one increases during the years just before, during and after the menopause. These observations constitute very strong evidence that by their presence, female sex hormones diminish—and by their absence, increase—vulnerability to ulcers. Take Molly's case, for example.

GLASGOW, SCOTLAND. AUGUST 27, 1976

Molly, a twenty-seven-year-old dance instructor and part-time hairdresser, has been married for four years and is childless. She and her husband have tried to avoid pregnancy because of the fear that Molly's ulcer, intermittently but frequently active since a year after they were married, would be made worse by the stress of raising a family. Nevertheless, Molly accidentally became pregnant seven months ago. A month after the baby was conceived, Molly's pain, previously never absent for more than a week or two at a time, disappeared.

Molly gives birth to a healthy baby girl in October. She decides to breast-feed the child. By the time the baby is six months old, Molly's ulcer symptoms have returned, slowly and mildly at first. Six months later Molly's ulcer is full-blown and active again. It seriously interferes with her life. Naturally disappointed and frustrated, she and her husband are now considering surgery in hopes of complete and permanent relief.

Studies on large groups of Scottish women with ulcers have shown that the menstrual cycle has no appreciable influence on either the development of new ulcers or the intensity of symptoms from existing ulcers. However, pregnancy brings relief from complaints almost 90 percent of the time. Women whose ulcer is inactive immediately before conceiving a child continue to be free from ulcer symptoms. In others the symptoms appear to clear up dramatically at an early stage of the pregnancy.

Unhappily, the benefits derived from pregnancy tend to be temporary. Almost half the women with ulcers whose symptoms disappear during pregnancy have a recurrence of their symptoms by the end of the third month after delivery. By the end of the sixth month after the baby's birth almost three-quarters of these women can expect to suffer recurrences. By the time the child is two years old, almost every one of these women will have had a flare-up of her ulcer. The recurrence of ulcer symptoms in women whose symptoms have disappeared during pregnancy is likely to occur even earlier following delivery if the mother lactates and the baby is breast-fed.

These observations support the notion that the female sex hormones, which are produced in large quantities during pregnancy, do in fact have a beneficial effect on the healing of ulcers. This has been corroborated in many ways. Here is an unusual example:

NAIROBI, KENYA. OCTOBER 26, 1955

Nnewaneka is a twenty-five-year-old black *male* South African native who along with nine other members of his tribe has been brought into the city by a missionary van; all are suffering from severe malnutrition. Two seasons of drought have destroyed consecutive crops and left the members of Nnewaneka's tribe living at near-starvation levels.

Nnewaneka is six feet six inches tall, weighs 115 pounds, and has long spindly arms and legs and a pot belly. His liver can easily be felt and is three times normal size, accounting in large part for his distended abdomen. His testicles are tiny and atrophied; his breasts are enlarged and resemble those of a normal fourteen-year-old girl.

Except for the poor nutritional status of these people, they're otherwise basically well. It's particularly noteworthy that none of the members of the tribe have stomach or duodenal ulcers. They, and others in similar circumstances, have been noted to have an especially low incidence of ulcer compared to the members of other tribes living further to the west, where the soil is richer and agriculture more productive and predictable. Even white settlers living in the same area as Nnewaneka and his tribe suffer from ulcers far more frequently.

What can a starving male South African black possibly have in common with a pregnant Caucasian Scotswoman? Interestingly, they share a remarkably similar hormonal state—Molly's as a natural consequence of her pregnancy, Nnewaneka's as a result of severe malnutrition. Diet probably plays an indirect role in the very *low* frequency of peptic ulcers observed in black South Africans. Malnourished Africans often have high blood levels of female sex hormones as a result of the starving liver's inability to metabolize them. Enlargement of the male breasts (gynecomastia) and small, atrophic testicles are features of elevated estrogens. These observations offer further evidence that female hormones may help protect against the development of ulcers.* The idea that female sex hormones may have a salutary effect in some predominantly male diseases is neither far-fetched nor new; coronary artery disease, as one example, affects many more men than women.

Of course pregnancy also involves changes other than those in hormone levels, and *these* may have a bearing on a woman's ulcer problem. Pregnant women are much more likely to pay close attention to what they eat and to take good

---

* During the early 1940's there was a surge of interest in the possibility of using female sex hormones to treat ulcers. In fact, beneficial effects were observed in a few controlled studies. But for the most part the results of other studies were disappointing, so the notion did not survive the test of time. Perhaps the doses of female hormones given did not, or could not, match the levels normally found in females during a natural pregnancy. Unfortunately, at present very little research on the relationship between ulcers and hormones seems to be going on.

care of themselves. Emotional and psychological factors may also contribute to a state of mental and physical well-being. Some women leave their job when they become pregnant, and (depending, of course, on how they feel about the job) this may eliminate one form of stress.

THE MENOPAUSE AND WOMEN WITH ULCER

Just as the high estrogen levels resulting from pregnancy may act as a balm for ulcers in women, the menopause seems to make women more vulnerable to them. In fact, as men and women move through their fifties, sixties and seventies, the gap between the incidence of ulcers in men and that in women grows smaller and smaller; it is never again as wide as it is during their thirties and forties.

Although too much acid is commonly thought of as a cause of ulcers, the incidence of new ulcers or the flare-up of already existing ones in menopausal women doesn't appear to be related to the levels of acid produced.* At all ages women tend to make less stomach acid than men, but low or

---

* In some experiments we performed in our own laboratories and reported in 1965, we noted that gastric-acid secretion doubled in female dogs when they were injected with testosterone, a long-acting male hormone. Acid secretion further doubled when the animal's ovaries were removed. Finally, when we stopped male hormone injections in the castrated dogs, acid levels fell but never returned to normal. We inferred from our study that male hormone factors may be aggressive, at least in terms of acid secretion, and could therefore possibly play a role in the production of ulcers, although none were found in these animals. We concluded that the ovaries, with their potential for the manufacture of female hormones, act as a "braking" or suppressing mechanism. Once they are removed, other as yet undetermined factors contribute to an increased acid production. These are interesting observations, but since we know that in post-menopausal woman acid secretion from the stomach is not especially elevated, the information does not provide us with the answers we seek.

absent acid secretion is *particularly* characteristic of women in the menopausal and post-menopausal age groups.

We know that with the diminution in female sex hormones during the menopause some mucous membranes such as those in the vagina secrete less fluid and atrophy. And since the mucous lining of the stomach, mouth, intestines and vagina have a great deal in common, this process of atrophy may explain why older women have more ulcers than younger ones. It's a giant step, however, to translate these observations into a clear-cut cause-and-effect relationship, and based on the data currently available I am reluctant to do so.

Of course during the menopause, whether it occurs naturally or is brought on by surgery, a woman may experience some loss of self-esteem. Or the general aging process may play a role entirely separate from that of hormonal change. Other factors such as the death of a spouse or the "empty nest" syndrome may also influence health and well-being. All of these factors may have some bearing on the increase in the incidence of ulcers in menopausal and post-menopausal women.

EMOTION, STRESS AND PERSONALITY FACTORS IN WOMEN WITH ULCERS

Unfortunately, most of the information dealing with the effects of emotions and personality in causing ulcers in women was accumulated many years ago, some of it dating as far back as the nineteenth century, when society was more a "man's world" than it is today. Still, even recent studies have a clear-cut sexist bias introduced by the fact that male physicians are evaluating female patients. In light of our current awareness of the many myths and misconceptions that have been perpetrated concerning abstract and often elusive "differences" between men and women, certainly the information needs reevaluation.

The writings on women with ulcers tend to emphasize psychosomatic factors * rather than physiological and hormonal
ones. An unusually heavy weight is often placed on feminine
emotion and the female psychology.† Women with ulcers are
still commonly described as being neurotic, emotionally disturbed and/or depressed; having severe character disorders;
suffering from low self-esteem; having high anxiety levels;
and so forth. These personality characteristics are believed
to be more prevalent in female than in male ulcer patients.
Consider, for example, the case of Suzanne.

PARIS, FRANCE. 7:15 A.M., SEPTEMBER 27, 1972

Suzanne is lying on an operating table. She is about to undergo surgery for a duodenal ulcer that has bled four times
in nine months. She's an attractive thirty-year-old heiress
and a successful fashion designer.

Acquaintances describe her as a hard-driving, strong-
willed woman. She wears her dark hair short, dresses only
in men's jeans, and treats her passive, rather shy husband as
an errand boy. Their two-year-old marriage is deeply trou-
bled. She repeatedly threatens to "throw him out and cut
him off without a cent."

Sue was perfectly healthy until shortly after her father,
an enormously successful politician, banker and inter-

---

* This is also true of the writings on men with ulcers, but the patterns that emerge are less well defined and consequently not stressed to
the same degree. This doesn't mean that the patterns aren't there, only
that they haven't been clearly delineated.

† In one study, for example, Indian women from a certain northwest
coastal tribe had a frequency of duodenal ulcer greater than that of
the male members of the tribe, and about four times greater than that
of non-Indian women in the United States. They developed ulcers at an
earlier age than the Indian men, and had an unusually high rate of
psychoneurotic and psycho-physiological disorders. The authors of this
study concluded that due to their vast family responsibility, these
women were under a great deal of psychological stress, and that they
therefore were more susceptible to developing ulcers.

national financier, died in the spring of 1971. Her parents have been divorced for more than eighteen years. For fourteen months the ulcer symptoms and repeated hospitalizations for pain and bleeding have made her domestic, social and professional life a nightmare. She has become increasingly disruptive of others' affairs, and demanding in her own. She wants what she wants when she wants it.

This operation is not the end of her troubles. Although her postoperative course will be uncomplicated, she will be dissatisfied with the results. She will have continuing complaints for the rest of her life.

At a 1951 meeting of the American Psychiatric Association, E. Kezur and his coworkers presented the results of a study in which twenty-five women with peptic ulcers were evaluated from the psychosomatic point of view. The characterizations were based on as much information as possible, some subjects undergoing up to three hundred psychiatric interviews *each*. Such other sources as relatives and social agencies were sometimes used to provide additional information.

Particular attention was paid to the relationships between the patient and her parents. As children, none of these women experienced a normal mother-child relationship. In many cases the mother had "spoiled" or rejected the patient, or died or deserted her at an early age.

In contrast, these women generally had a closer, more satisfying and more positive relationship to their father. Many of these women identified with male figures, this identification often surfacing in "tomboy" traits and subsequently in marriage to passive men. Hostile feelings toward men or fear of them and poor sexual adjustment were also very common. Often patients were both passive and aggressive.

In almost all of the women the onset or aggravation of ulcer symptoms occurred in conjunction with the death of, or rejection or desertion by, a husband or fiancé. Ulcer symptoms arose in some patients when their father or (in two cases) both parents died or were "lost."

Such findings are often reported by those who have studied women with ulcers. They have been interpreted as illustrating a "dependent" need which these women meet by a denial of reality. The pattern of an early loss of a mother figure either by death or rejection and a subsequent identification with the father or (later on) the husband crops up frequently. Subsequent collapse of the relationship with the male figure to whom identification has been transferred, or failure on the part of the male to properly assume the "identity role," may then lead to the onset or aggravation of ulcer symptoms.

Other studies seem to corroborate at least some of this. In 1967, M. L. Pilot and his coworkers at Yale reported on an extensive study and psychiatric evaluation they had done of forty-one women with duodenal ulcers. They also found a relatively high incidence of physical loss of or desertion by the patient's mother (eleven cases) and father (eight cases) prior to her achieving sexual maturity. Just before the onset of ulcer disease many of these patients experienced either a loss of, or difficulty with, some person closely associated to them, often their husband. The second most common loss was that of a child; the third, that of a patient's mother. A number of patients suffered multiple losses. Finally, the married patients often had husbands with problems: among these men, psychosis, severe medical illnesses and alcoholism were common. In some cases the patients were widowed.

Interestingly, although many of the patients worked, in only one case were ulcer symptoms related to difficulty with a boss or employer. Many of these women seemed to be capable, independent and openly self-reliant. Still, at the time of the onset of symptoms, almost all experienced some sort of change in their emotional defense mechanisms. According to the Yale researchers, this pattern was different from that of men with ulcers. Women with ulcer often expressed a deep feeling of disappointment, "as though [they] had expected something from the love object and had been surprised not to find or experience it."

Attempts have been made to seek still other precipitating factors in the lives of women with ulcers. For example, consider Sarah's case:

LARCHMONT, NEW YORK. FEBRUARY 28, 1974

A fifty-eight-year-old socially active and community-spirited housewife, Sarah is the mother of three grown sons. Her husband is sixty-four and hopes to sell his successful lumberyard and building-contract business next year. They expect to retire to Phoenix or Palm Springs and enjoy life.

Sarah's been basically well all her life except for a bout with duodenal ulcer fifteen years earlier, during a marital crisis. After seven months of intensive therapy it healed and lay dormant for almost fourteen years.

In 1972 Sarah's uterus, Fallopian tubes, and ovaries were removed because of uterine fibroid tumors and spotting of blood from her vagina. She had no trouble with the surgery, but six months after it was done, her ulcer kicked up quite suddenly. She's having a very difficult time controlling it with medications. It has bled once, slightly, though no transfusions were required. Sarah and her husband are considering surgery for her ulcer so that they can enjoy their retirement unmarred by health problems.

Some gynecologic surgery, particularly procedures in which the woman is sterilized, may frequently be followed by psycho-physiological gastrointestinal reactions. In 1956 S. I. Cohen, A. J. Silverman and F. Magnusson reported that one-quarter of a group of 200 female ulcer patients they'd studied had been sterilized just prior to developing ulcer symptoms. Another fifth of this group had undergone a major gynecologic procedure, and another quarter of them had become menopausal. In almost 70 percent of the subjects studied, therefore, it was possible to identify an event that, according to the authors, consciously or unconsciously threatened the patient's sexual functions or her "identity as a woman."

The investigators also felt that they could identify some

clear-cut personality characteristics among these women. Some of the women were aggressive and rejected the "female role" (as defined by society). Some felt inadequate and had difficulty adapting to what are traditionally considered adult responsibilities. In this group as well, the death or loss of a supporting figure was a prominent feature in the onset of symptoms. The largest subgroup of these women had accepted the traditional female role and seemed to function well until they had major gynecologic surgery leading to sterilization, or experienced the onset of menopause.

The personality and emotional traits supposedly characteristic of women with ulcers have consistently been corroborated by many sources and deserve careful consideration. Of course there are many exceptions to these characterizations, though many of these features *are* commonly seen. Many terms that appear again and again throughout the studies—such words, for example, as aggressiveness, passivity, hostility, fearfulness, masculinity, dependency, or inadequacy —are obviously subjective ones, the application of which is very dependent on the particular observer. Other observations are quite concrete—the effects of pregnancy and the menopause (natural or surgical), the remarkable frequency with which ulcer symptoms first appear or reappear following divorce, loss of a child, loss of a mate or parent, or surgical procedures on female sex organs. Unfortunately, however, almost all of the descriptions of personality and emotional features of women with ulcers are based on data from very small population samples and often inadequate control groups.

Be that as it may, there is ample evidence that ulcers in women are very different from ulcers in men.

10

Ulcers in Children

It is customary, but I think it is a mistake to speak of happy childhood. Children, however, are often over-anxious and acutely sensitive. Man ought to be man and master of his fate; but children are at the mercy of those around them.
—Sir John Lubdock (1834–1913)

The childhood shews the man,
As morning shews the day.
—John Milton (1608–1674),
Paradise Regained

Even the most devoted and loving parents find it hard to appreciate the stresses home, school and social environments place on youngsters. Mothers and fathers, their own lives full of obligations, conflicts and anxieties, sometimes forget that children also have deeply felt emotions of their own. Relationships with teachers, classmates and friends; the need to succeed academically or socially; goals to be set and achieved; even financial problems—all contribute to a world as pressured as an adult's. Also, a child detects and responds to friction in parental relationships, so a great deal of anxiety may be transmitted from parent to child. Not only are children at the mercy of the environment, but simple immaturity and lack of experience make it harder for them to cope with the stress at hand.

Who knows whether or not the twentieth-century child is as able to cope with the world as children who marched in the Crusades? Or whether scavenging for food in Bangladesh is more or less stressful than fumbling an infield grounder in a Little League ball game. I do know however, that children are keenly aware of, and profoundly affected by, what goes on around them, far more than we give them credit for.

Bela Schick, the developer of the Schick test for diptheria, once said that children are not simply micro-adults, but have their own special problems. Ulcers may well be one of them. Unfortunately the remarkable scarcity of medical literature on the subject of children with ulcers wrongly suggests that such cases are rare and relatively unimportant. True, ulcers are basically a problem of adulthood: the most common age of onset is sometime between sixteen and twenty-five. Actually, most people who get ulcers tend to be even older at the time the disorder begins. But cases of children with ulcers are far more common than we had previously thought.

There's a definite tendency to underdiagnose this condition by both parents and doctors, partly because the clinical features of the child's disorder are frequently atypical of the adult's, and partly because parents and physicians are quite naturally reluctant to subject children to extensive laboratory and x-ray examinations. Abdominal pain is very common in children of all ages, and the conditions that usually account for it are far more ordinary than ulcers; as a result the possibility of ulcers may not be considered often enough. This unwillingness or inability to *think* of ulcers as a possible cause of abdominal pain in children may well have contributed to its apparent rarity.

Ulcers in children aren't all that rare. Over a sixteen-year period in a Wisconsin clinic, 337 children with ulcers were discovered. According to another study from Erie County, New York, the number of cases recognized by doctors increased from 1 in 200,000 children during the period from 1947 to 1949 to 8 in 200,000 during the 1956 to 1958 period. Although the investigators acknowledged that this increase could be due to greater awareness of the disorder and better diagnostic techniques, they hypothesized that increasing psychological pressures on children could also be involved. In any event, ulcers *are* an important health problem in children, and increasing numbers of cases have been reported from clinics in widely separated geographic locations throughout the world. Since about 2 percent of adults with ulcers can trace the onset of their abdominal complaints back to childhood, the numbers of youngsters who currently suffer from the disorder can be estimated to be many thousands in the United States alone.

Linda is a fairly typical example of a youngster with duodenal ulcer:

SACRAMENTO, CALIFORNIA. AUGUST 5, 1972

Linda is a nine-and-a-half-year-old Chinese American girl. Her father, with whom she lives, and her mother, who has returned to her hometown of Seattle, were recently divorced. Her father suffers from an ulcer.

For the past two months she's been plagued by frequent headaches, nausea, abdominal pain and occasional vomiting. Despite his own experience with stomach troubles her dad attributes her complaints to "the kind of bellyache all kids complain of from time to time." Although she has a good school record, the quality of her work has deteriorated. She's finally taken to a doctor.

Quiet, withdrawn and somewhat depressed, she submitted to physical examination without complaint. Her stomach was x-rayed and an active ulcer crater was noted in the first portion of the duodenum. A bland diet and acid-neutralizing drugs were prescribed, and psychotherapy was recommended.

Her symptoms disappeared, and she enjoyed a long period of freedom from discomfort. Two years later, however, while preparing for an important school test, she complained of severe upper abdominal pain, sudden in onset. She was rushed to the hospital, where x-rays of her abdomen revealed the presence of free air under the diaphragm. She was taken to the operating room, where a hole in the duodenum caused by a perforated ulcer was found and repaired.

She did well for eighteen months, but then after a prolonged visit with her mother she once again was tormented by abdominal pain and began to pass black tarry stools. She was again admitted to the hospital, where a blood transfusion was deemed necessary; further surgery for "definitive" control of her ulcer was recommended. Three days later she underwent an operation in which the vagus nerves to her stomach were cut and the pyloric outlet enlarged. There were no complications, and she remains well up to the present.

Although ulcers in children are similar in many respects to ulcers in adults, there are some interesting differences. For example, the gap between the number of male children who get ulcers and the number of female children who do is far less pronounced than it is in adults. Adult males with ulcers sometimes outnumber females with ulcers ten to one, but in children the distribution between the sexes varies from equality to only somewhat higher—about three boys to each girl. This relatively low predominance of male children with ulcers is a fairly constant observation and has been reported from clinics in such widely separated places as Belfast, Pittsburgh, India and Nigeria. In one study the ratio was actually reversed, girls outnumbering boys 139 to 125. As was mentioned in Chapter 9, these observations may offer a clue to the role of sex hormones in either causing or protecting against ulcers, a factor that may not come into full play until after the age of sexual maturity.

Children with ulcers often come from families in which

one or more members have the disorder. A family history of the ailment exists in up to 65 percent of such cases. Sometimes the mother and occasionally both parents suffer from ulcer, but usually the father is the "carrier"—in fact, in up to one-third of the cases. In any event, the most frequently affected kin are those that are most closely related to the children: parents, brothers and sisters. These are extraordinary findings; not only are they consistent with the data normally reported for adults, but they outstrip it. Parents and physicians should definitely consider the possibility of ulcers in cases of children with abdominal pain who also have a family history of the disorder.

These patterns suggest that there are genetically determined factors which, just as in the adult, may play a role in the causation of ulcers in children. The importance of heredity is further emphasized by the fact that, as in adults, a significantly higher than normal percentage of youngsters with the disease belong to blood group type O. Naturally, common environmental influences within the family can't be ruled out.

This strong tendency for several members of the same family to develop ulcers also signals the possibility that a common stressful environment may have something to do with their development. And indeed, instability in the home may be a dominant contributing factor. However, both "stress" and "instability" are elusive terms, difficult to interpret precisely. Tension, anxiety, perfectionism and phobias do seem to occur in varying degrees in children with ulcers. Up to one in four may have serious emotional problems. According to some studies, almost 40 percent of children affected with ulcers had parents of different religious backgrounds, while only about one in ten children with chronic diseases other than ulcers came from mixed marriages.

That a child with ulcers is under great emotional stress at home and/or in school seems to be a very common observation. A deterioration in the relationship between the parents has been noted in almost four times as many families in which there are children with ulcers as families in which there are children with other serious illnesses.

All of us can learn something from this information. In their recently published book *Open Family Living,* Thomas McGinnis and John Ayres have pointed out that people commonly treat each other in ways they originally learned in their families when they were children. Individuals who have gentle and considerate parents may find it natural to behave with gentleness and consideration. The child of angry, violent parents often feels more at home with anger and violence. Children of indifferent, neglectful parents may become alienated and often have trouble establishing any kind of intimate human relationships. A clue to the prevention of ulcers in children may possibly be found in these sensible observations.

As far as acid is concerned, as with adults, an extremely wide range in variation of levels can be found among youngsters of similar ages and general state of health. However, there does not seem to be a reliable pattern in children with ulcers. In fact, some researchers have observed that most youngsters with the ailment have either normal or somewhat low acid outputs. Based on the information we now have available, the levels of acid secretion in children with ulcers has not been absolutely defined as a consistent diagnostic feature. It may even be true that the presence in the stomach of large amounts of hydrochloric acid and pepsin may not be as critical to the development of ulcers in children as in adults. Such other factors as defective or immature defense mechanisms may be at play. This, however, is only speculation.

Children often complain of belly pain, and innumerable conditions can account for it, most of which occur far more frequently than do ulcers. Bellyache is nevertheless the single most important symptom of ulcers. So while I have no desire to alarm you in every situation in which your child complains of a bellyache, here are some of the more characteristic complaints of children with ulcers.

Most children with ulcers point to the area around the belly button as the source of their pain. Others tend to report that it is situated in the middle upper abdomen. Ulcer pain tends to occur with about equal frequency in boys and girls. This pain tends to be intermittent and periodic, sometimes disappearing entirely for days or weeks at a time. For many children food has no effect on the pain. For others, about as many claim that eating intensifies the pain as say that eating relieves it. The relationship of ulcer symptoms with food is therefore not very helpful in making the diagnosis.

Pain at night, even to the point of awakening the child, is another common feature of ulcers in children. The next most common symptoms are nausea and vomiting, which often occur immediately after or even during a meal. Surprisingly, considering the fact that peptic ulcer is a disorder of the gastrointestinal tract, children with ulcers don't seem to complain about changes in bowel habits, nor have such changes been noticed by parents or physicians.

Children with peptic ulcer have an inordinately high incidence of such complications as bleeding or perforation, possibly because the diagnosis of ulcers may not be arrived at until complications actually develop. Often there's a long lag between the actual onset of the disorder and the point at which it is recognized by either the parents or the physician. This, of course, is especially true of peptic ulcer that begins in the newborn.

In very young children or infants under the age of two, the complications of hemorrhage and perforation commonly occur together with or following a major illness such as meningitis or some other severe infection. Needless to say, in these tiny patients such complications are extremely serious, and the mortality rate is very high. Perforation of the duodenum or stomach in these youngsters is especially common and lethal. Some factors that may play a role in causing ulcer in children of this age group include brain damage, infection, major injuries, congenital or hereditary weakness in the muscles of the stomach, major burns, and congenital heart disease.

MEDICAL TREATMENT OF CHILDREN WITH ULCERS

The general feeling in the medical community is that peptic ulcers in children tend to heal spontaneously. Yet considering the high complication rate and the fact that retrospective studies show that at least 2 percent of adults with ulcers have symptoms that began in childhood, this is probably an overly optimistic attitude. In fact the long-term success rate for managing ulcers in children by medication alone is not even as high as the success rate for adults.

More than half of children who suffer from peptic ulcer, in comparison to only 10 or 15 percent of adults with the disorder, ultimately require surgery. Still, an intense medically oriented program of therapy should be tried first. Such a regimen should include supervision of the child's diet and the prescription of acid-neutralizing and -controlling medications. Psychotherapy and family counseling should be considered. Finally, during the acute phase of an ulcer flare-up in children, it's often helpful to have the child drink milk on an hourly basis in conjunction with taking the acid-controlling drugs.

It's especially difficult to evaluate this sort of treatment in children. The rhythmicity and periodicity of ulcer, with periods of healing alternating with periods of flare-up, makes it almost impossible to differentiate between ulcers that are healing spontaneously and those that are truly responding to therapy. Barring complications, however, medication and diet should be tried, and your physician's recommendations should be followed diligently. The only alternative is surgery.

SURGERY FOR CHILDREN WITH ULCERS

Ulcer patients of all ages require surgery when such complications as massive vomiting of blood or passage of blood in the stools, perforation of the ulcer, obstruction of the stomach's outlet, and uncontrollable pain develop. Although intractability (when an ulcer does not heal even with medication) is the most common reason for operating on adults with ulcers, hemorrhage and perforation seem to be more frequent precipitating factors in children. It may be, however, that an intractable ulcer in a child too young to express complaints clearly is ignored or overlooked. When a child tells you he or she has abdominal pain, while the cause may be nothing more serious than constipation or too many green apples, pay attention.

The elements involved in the choice of a specific type of operation for an adult ulcer patient should probably also be considered in the case of a child. Your physician and surgeon will naturally give you the best advice possible based on their own experience. Some doctors have recommended that surgery done on children be as conservative as possible, and simply cutting the vagus nerves and enlarging the outlet of the stomach has been the treatment most often used. In Chapter 14 some of these operations will be discussed in greater detail.

I consider the early age of onset of peptic ulcers in children to indicate the particular virulence of this disease. I believe that management of ulcers in youngsters should probably be more aggressive. We do know that a conservative removal of a small portion of the stomach combined with the cutting of the vagus nerves effects a cure in almost 100 percent of the cases. Studies done on puppies indicate that this operation does not affect growth and development. Our experience with children indicates that this operation ("resective" procedures in which less than half the stomach is removed) does not appear to interfere with the nutritional status or growth patterns of children so treated. A high percentage do very well.

But surgery done on children with ulcers has a significant mortality rate, probably because many of these operations are performed on an emergency basis. When the surgery is done electively on a planned and carefully thought out basis, rather than as an emergency procedure in the middle of the night, the mortality rate should be very low—indeed, comparable to the rate for adults. For this reason, undue delay of effective treatment should not be permitted.

III

THE DIAGNOSIS AND TREATMENT OF ULCERS

11

Ulcer Symptoms and Diagnosis

You cannot be sure of the success of your remedy, while you
are still uncertain of the nature of the disease.
—Peter Mere Latham (1789–1875),
Diseases of the Heart, Lecture XIV

In America about one in every ten men and one in every
twenty women. will develop ulcers sometime during their
life. That's a lot of people with ulcers. Somewhere around
10 million men and 5 million women alive today have or
will have a peptic ulcer.

From time to time all of us suffer some form of abdominal
pain; you may call it indigestion, gas pains, sour stomach,
heartburn, hunger pains, morning-after stomach, or some
other name. But many people then decide, without benefit of
medical counsel, that because they have abdominal pain,
they either have or are going to develop ulcers. These same
people often begin to treat themselves with one or another

of the widely advertised remedies for "stomach distress." Sales of over-the-counter stomach medications, even as long as ten years ago, exceed $80,000,000 a year.

The first step in the treatment of peptic ulcer should be unequivocal establishment of the diagnosis. It's foolish and potentially dangerous to simply leap to the conclusion that you have an ulcer and then treat yourself with over-the-counter antacid preparations. Your symptoms could be caused by something unrelated to your stomach or duodenum; moreover, *another* disorder—one perhaps even more serious than ulcers—may be present. If you suffer from abdominal symptoms that persist for more than a few days, if you think you have an ulcer, or if you have had an ulcer that feels like it is now kicking up, seek the advice of a competent physician. Your problem will then be as much his as yours. You'll be well rewarded by relief from anxiety and by a prompt and properly oriented attack on whatever you have, be it ulcers or not.

YOUR HISTORY

Your history is the single most important and persuasive element in properly diagnosing your condition. Naturally, the newborn infant, the small child, the extremely elderly, or the person with a language barrier must rely on others to present an orderly and sequential story of their complaints. But the way you tell your story can have an influence on how fast and effectively your doctor can deal with your disorder.

Before you visit your physician it's sometimes helpful to make a few notes—perhaps even to consult with your spouse or other members of your family—in order to refresh your own memory of events so that you can present your history concisely and clearly. Here's a guide to the sort of thing your physician will want to know.

Who You Are and What Your Chief Complaint Is: Start out by telling your physician your age and the type of work you do. Then begin with your chief complaint.

Be sure to tell him where the pains were when they began and what circumstances surrounded their onset. Describe the pain—is it stabbing, burning, gnawing, pressure-like, or something else? Characterize the intensity of the complaint, using such terms as "excruciating," "mild" or "moderate."

Are the pains constant or are they intermittent—and if intermittent, what is the length of time between attacks? Do they always begin in the same place and stay there, or do they radiate to other parts of your abdomen, back or chest? How long do they last? Can you identify anything that brings the pains on or relieves them? Do you have night pain, and are you awakened by it? Are the attacks getting more frequent and more severe, are they staying at about the same level, or are they more moderate and less frequent, with longer periods of freedom from pain?

Does activity or the position in which your body is placed affect the kind of pain you are having? (That is, does lying down or getting up and walking around help or make the pain worse?)

Last, since the pain seems to center about your gastrointestinal tract, do you have other related problems besides pain? Have you been vomiting? Do you feel gassy or bloated after eating? Have your bowel habits changed? Is constipation or diarrhea a new feature? Do you notice blood in your stools? Have they changed in color? Has your weight changed in the past year?

Past History: Here you will want to tell the physician about any operations you may have had in the past, and any injuries or childhood diseases (for example, measles, mumps, chicken pox or pneumonia). Also, mention any serious illnesses and hospitalizations you may have had—heart disease, kidney disease, disease of the lungs, disease in your urinary tract or genitals, diabetes, tuberculosis, and so on.

Family History: Are your parents still living? If they are, what is their state of health? If they are not, what did they die of? Did they have any serious illnesses? Did they have ulcers? How about your brothers and sisters? Their medical histories will also be of interest to your physician.

Smoking, Alcohol and Other Drinking Habits, Diet and Medications: Do you smoke? How much alcohol do you drink in the course of a week? How much coffee or tea do you drink per day? Are you taking any drugs or medications of any kind? *Be sure to include a history of aspirin-taking.*

What is your diet like? Do you eat three full meals a day? Do you snack? Has your weight changed in the last year? If so, why do you think it has? Are you dieting or overeating? Are there any special foods that bother you? Are there particular foods that you avoid or that you crave? Do some foods seem to help your pain? Do some make it worse?

Organ Systems Review: Here you may want to tell the physician that you have or have not had any trouble with your brain or central nervous system, your eyes, ears, nose or throat, your heart or lungs, your liver, gallbladder, pancreas, and bowels; mention any urinary-tract disorders you may have had, such as bladder infections or prostate trouble. If you're female, tell him your menstrual history, how many pregnancies you've had, and how many children you have. You will also want to tell him how your arms and legs work and whether you can or cannot put in a full day's work without any particular problems. You will want to give him a sexual history as well. Finally, you must be sure to tell him about any previous operations or injuries and/or any other things you may feel are pertinent to the story of your general physical and emotional being—*as you see it.*

This seems like a lot to tell the doctor, but don't be afraid of taking up too much of his time or boring him. His problems will be simplified by a *concise* and *orderly* history. He'll question you at greater length on certain facets of your history, and if you start to stray from what he really wants to know, he will let you know. Try to minimize unrelated or conversational aspects of your history. The whole business of relating your health problems to him can be accomplished in five to ten minutes by some preparation on your part and skill on his. Often, based on your personal history alone, he can begin to formulate some idea of what your problem is. The physical examination that follows will be more efficient if he knows where to look more carefully, although on your first visit he may want to examine you from head to toe.

Only then will he mention what sort of diagnostic procedures are required to pinpoint the problem and suggest how you and he can go about arranging for them. He may at this point even offer you a tentative diagnosis.

ULCER PAIN

The single most consistent thread in the fabric which makes up the diagnosis of ulcer is pain. Although there can be many other complaints, the abdominal discomfort usually drives the patient to seek medical advice. The specific character of ulcer pain can strongly suggest the proper diagnosis in a significant percentage of people. Take Lars's story as an example:

MINNEAPOLIS, MINNESOTA. JANUARY 26, 1976

Lars is a forty-four-year-old Caucasian customer relations officer at a major bank. His symptoms date back approximately two and a half years. In the spring of 1974 he noticed a gnawing, boring pain that generally appeared between one and four hours after a meal and was localized in the upper mid-abdomen just below the lowest level of the breastbone, approximately four inches above his navel and slightly to the right. This pain normally lasts between half an hour and one and a half hours, and it can be relieved by the ingestion of milk or food. When Lars is having an "attack," the pain comes daily for a period of two to three weeks. The attack is followed by a period of freedom from symptoms that may last weeks or even months.

Lars rarely feels the pain before breakfast. The onset is somewhat later, often during the period from nine to ten-thirty in the morning when he is just settling down to work. The morning pain is sometimes more cramp-like than gnawing and boring in nature. Other times it is more burning or aching in nature. The pain may last for only twenty minutes to an hour, after which it may spontaneously disappear. Or it may persist until medication or eating something brings relief.

Lars rarely has pain that awakes him in the middle of the night unless he also has symptoms in the evening before retiring. Although the evening pain may be relieved by food, it quite often recurs sometime between midnight and 2:00 A.M. If just prior to retiring, he has taken a snack, the evening pain, when it occurs at all, may develop somewhat later.

Lars rarely becomes nauseated, and he has never vomited as a result of this disorder. To his surprise, his appetite has remained good. Still, he's lost about ten pounds over the last year. This can be attributed to his reluctance to eat full meals for fear, paradoxically, of initiating his discomfort.

When his symptoms first appeared, the periods of freedom between attacks lasted six to ten weeks. Of late they have been coming after increasingly shorter intervals. Discomfort has been more severe and is less responsive to both food and medication. Lars has most of the common characteristics of pain arising from duodenal ulcer.

Nausea and vomiting are not very common symptoms of duodenal ulcers. When these symptoms do appear, it is usually when the outlet of the stomach (pylorus) is partly obstructed by the ulcer scar or inflammation and the stomach can't completely empty itself. They may also occur without obstruction, but usually not unless pain is also present.

There are some basic differences between the pain of duodenal ulcer and that of gastric ulcer. In the latter the pain tends to be less intermittent and more persistent. Also, whereas the pain of duodenal ulcer usually occurs between meals, gastric ulcer pains may begin during or right after a meal. Eating is much less likely to relieve the symptoms of a gastric ulcer patient, and it may even aggravate them.

ULCER PAIN

DUODENAL	GASTRIC
RELATIVELY INTERMITTENT	RELATIVELY CONSTANT
ONSET BETWEEN MEALS OR WHEN STOMACH IS EMPTY	MAY BEGIN WITH OR SOON AFTER MEALS
FOOD OFTEN RELIEVES SYMPTOMS	FOOD LESS LIKELY TO RELIEVE SYMPTOMS
MID-ABDOMINAL IN LOCATION, JUST BELOW BREASTBONE	OFTEN MID-ABDOMINAL AND SLIGHTLY TO THE LEFT
MAY BORE THROUGH TO THE BACK	BACK PAIN RARE

The pain of both duodenal and gastric ulcers occurs in the upper mid-abdomen, but the pain of the gastric ulcer is commonly somewhat to the left. Although duodenal ulcer pain may bore through to your back, such pain is rare with gastric ulcer. On the other hand, nausea, bloating, vomiting and burping are much more common with gastric ulcer.

Thus the pain you are suffering may be the most prominent characteristic of an ulcer, and a careful description of it most helpful to your physician.

THE CAUSE OF ULCER PAIN

Pain is very subjective. It can't be felt or seen by the examining physician; an x-ray or telescopic examination of the stomach provides no indication of the degree of the discomfort. Its intensity varies not only from person to person but from time to time in the same individual. For example, a busy person absorbed in a particular project may be less aware of discomfort than someone who has a lot of time on his hands.

We don't know precisely why ulcers cause pain, although research has shown that acid bathing the raw surface of the ulcer may be the link. Swollen and inflamed tissues are definitely more sensitive to pain caused by acid. Most people with ulcers secrete acid on a relatively continuous basis between meals, but most ulcer pain lasts only two to four hours regardless of whether one does or does not eat or take neutralizing agents. Why then, if the acid secretion is continuous, isn't the pain continuous as well? Other factors besides acid must also play a role.

Hunger pains are basically different from ulcer pain in that they come and go quickly and are sometimes crampy. We really don't know much about what causes hunger pains except that they seem to be related to muscular contractions by the empty stomach. In contrast to true hunger pains, ulcer pain tends to be relatively steady, of low intensity, and aching or burning in nature.

X-RAY DIAGNOSIS

While your case history may indicate that it's likely you have a peptic ulcer, most physicians suggest that a few more precise and objective studies be done in order to be sure about the diagnosis. Such tests help the doctor differentiate between gastric and duodenal ulcers and also between benign and cancerous ones. Tests also assist the physician in checking for some other disorders that sometimes closely mimic ulcers—such as, for example, gallbladder disease, hiatus hernia, pancreatitis, outlet obstruction of the stomach from polyps or cancers (tumor), diverticuli (out-pouchings) of the upper gastrointestinal tract or the colon, gastritis (simple inflammation of the stomach without ulceration), inflammatory diseases of the small or large bowel, and even appendicitis.

The most valuable objective technique for determining whether or not ulcers are present is the barium x-ray study. The patient swallows a small amount of a chalklike dye that shows up on x-rays as a clear or white area; x-rays can reveal the structure of the esophagus, stomach, duodenum, small bowel and colon in remarkable detail. Evidence of leakage or perforation of the ulcer may also be noted.

This technique is safe as well as valuable. Furthermore, the patient feels very little discomfort during the procedure. However, accuracy is not perfect, and for a variety of reasons about 5 to 10 percent of ulcers may be missed by x-ray. Nevertheless, every patient in whom the diagnosis of peptic ulcer is being seriously considered *must* have such a study.

The combination of a strongly suggestive ulcer history and objective evidence of ulcer disease by x-ray may be all the confirmation your physician needs to begin treatment. Furthermore, a baseline is established so that the progress of therapy can be measured by repeating the x-ray study from time to time until it is obvious that the ulcer has completely healed.

ANALYSIS OF GASTRIC JUICES

Determining the rate at which you make acid may be helpful in diagnosing and treating ulcer for any or all of the following reasons:

1. A baseline is established by which the results of medical and surgical therapy can be evaluated in the future.

2. Knowing the amount of acid your stomach produces may help your doctor choose the proper medication or may help the surgeon "tailor" any operation you may have to your specific needs.

3. If your stomach doesn't make acid even in response to stimulation, a more thorough search for cancer must be carried out.

4. Rare endocrine disorders characterized by a tremendous overproduction of acid may be picked up by secretory analysis.

5. Some measure of the severity of the ulcer can be gained.

Not all physicians think stomach secretion studies are necessary or valuable. Statistical tables of normal acid secretory levels, based on the patient's age and sex, are helpful in determining whether any given subject is making normal, greater than normal, or less than normal amounts. The information that you produce far less or far more than normal amounts of acid can be helpful, but if your acid levels are in what is essentially the normal range the gastric secretory studies become less helpful. About 25 percent of the population make so much acid that they clearly have or will have peptic ulcer. At the other end of the scale, about 25 percent make so little acid that duodenal ulcer can probably be ruled out, although gastric ulcer may still be a possibility. There are so many exceptions to the rule, though, that secretory studies alone are almost never diagnostic of ulcers. They are mainly *helpful* in assessing the overall problem.

The method for studying gastric secretion is quite simple and safe, although probably a little more uncomfortable than the barium x-ray. You won't be allowed to eat or drink after midnight on the night before your examination. All drugs and medications that may have an effect on stomach secretion will also be discontinued well in advance. On the morning of the study you will be seated in a comfortable chair; then a fine tube will be passed through your nostril and into the stomach. While this may seem unpleasant, in the hands of a skillful physician or technician it is smoothly carried out. The tube should be located in the lowest portion of the stomach to ensure that all the gastric juice is collected and little or none escapes through the stomach outlet; your physician or the technician will take a quick x-ray to be sure that the tube is properly placed.

The stomach is completely emptied of all juices; these are measured and then discarded. Subsequent techniques vary from physician to physician, but in general two characteristics of gastric secretion are then evaluated.

Basal Acid Secretion:

The term "basal" implies that no environmental stimuli are affecting the rate of acid secretion. While it's impossible to completely eliminate all external factors, you will be put as completely at ease as possible. No loud noises or other threatening environmental factors will be permitted to reach you. The doctor cannot, however, eliminate your thought processes or other *internal* influences on stomach-acid secretion, but physicians accept this as a limitation of the study. As a matter of fact, these influences are among the things we wish to evaluate, for internal influences have a profound effect on acid secretion.

Despite the limitations of basal secretory studies and the inconsistency in the results, it's known that most people with duodenal ulcers make normal or greater than normal amounts of acid in the "resting" state, while people with gastric ulcers will usually make normal or less than normal amounts of acid.

Maximal Acid Output:

After the first hour, during which time the basal output is

established, you'll be injected with a stomach-acid stimulant. The maximal amount of acid you are capable of secreting in response to the stimulant is a far more reproducible piece of information than the basal secretory output. There is an almost linear relationship between the number of cells capable of making acid and the amount of acid produced by a stimulant. On different days and at different times during the same day, your peak acid output will vary by only a few percent.

Again, acid secretory studies are safe, although the stimulant used may produce some temporary side effects. However, these disappear quickly—within an hour or so in most instances—and do not represent a serious problem.

Exotic Secretory Studies:

Still other secretory studies are sometimes used to determine whether or not the vagus nerves are intact or have been successfully cut by surgery (see Chapter 14). These studies involve the use of insulin or some other agent known to stimulate the vagal centers in the brain, and are not used nearly to the extent that the basal and maximal secretory studies are.

TELESCOPIC (ENDOSCOPIC) EXAMINATION

The first medical instruments designed to examine some of the less accessible organs date from the early nineteenth century, when wax candles enclosed in a shaped tin tube were used. The earliest instruments used for examination of hollow organs were designed for use in the urinary bladder. It wasn't until 1881, the same year that the famous Viennese surgeon C. A. Theodor Billroth performed the first surgical removal of the stomach, that the "gastroscope" or stomach telescope was first introduced into medical practice. Rudimentary as the instrument was, it offered physicians the first real opportunity to see the inside of the stomach in a living human. By the turn of the twentieth century, cocaine and morphine were used as local anesthetics and sedatives and it was no longer necessary to put people to sleep for the examination. This increased the safety of the procedure and made it much more practical to use on the nonhospitalized person. These instruments improved yearly, and today they are so sophisticated that in experienced hands they are extremely safe and can provide views of the inside of the esophagus, stomach and duodenum that rival examination by the naked eye.

Diagnostic endoscopy of the upper gastrointestinal tract is also safe and very well tolerated. The risk involved in this type of examination is greater than the risk of either x-ray or acid studies, but in the hands of a skilled and experienced endoscopist the potential value far outweighs the dangers. I equate the exam with having a dental cavity filled. You will be sedated, sometimes enough to make you drowsy. You're not put to sleep because it's helpful to have your cooperation; the sedated but conscious subject is far easier to evaluate. The back of your throat will be anesthetized by a fine spray of local anesthesia so that you will be less aware of the passage of the telescope.

The telescope is as thick as your thumb, but is very flexible and can easily be tied in a knot. It will be passed gently through the back of your mouth into the upper esophagus, and from there down into your stomach and through the stomach into the duodenum. During this passage all of these areas will be carefully examined for evidence of disease. By means of cleverly placed channels incorporated into the body of the telescope, water can be injected to disperse debris that may be obscuring the examiner's vision, or suction can be applied to clear the juices from an area.

A camera attachment permits the examiner to photograph

any abnormality and to make the photo a part of your permanent medical record. It is even possible to add another flexible eyepiece so that two examiners can simultaneously view the tissues under study and can compare notes. If the need arises, a long biopsy instrument with a tip about the size of a grain of rice may be passed through the telescope, and a fragment of tissue can be taken for examination under a microscope.

Although it sounds complicated, endoscopy is now practiced in many, if not most, community hospitals throughout the United States. Though not an *essential* part of the diagnostic examination, it's often *desirable*. Take Eloise's case, for example.

ST. LOUIS, MISSOURI. 7:45 A.M., APRIL 17, 1977

Eloise is a fifty-three-year-old widowed lady with a gastric ulcer, established by x-ray the day before yesterday. Because of the ulcer's relatively unusual location on the greater curve of the stomach and because her stomach seems to make very little acid even when stimulated, her doctor is concerned about the possibility of tumor.

Eloise has had nothing to eat since yesterday evening and no liquids since midnight. Her medications were all given at their usual time, as they won't interfere with the endoscopy she is about to undergo.

Eloise is remarkably calm, although when the telescopic procedure was explained to her she was apprehensive. She has been given a sedative, which has made her drowsy, but she is quite cooperative. She is hooked up to an intravenous unit, and if necessary she can be sedated further—even put to sleep.

The endoscopist explains the instrument to her and tells her what he plans to do. First he'll spray the back of her throat to make it numb. He'll wait a few minutes and then spray it again. He'll place a bite block, a kind of plastic doughnut, between her teeth so she can comfortably close her mouth without damaging her teeth or the delicate instrument that will be passed in through the hole in the block.

While she's sitting up, the endoscope will be passed into her mouth, throat and upper esophagus. She will be asked to swallow as best as she can to help the lubricated instrument along. It passes through easily. Her endoscopist has done it hundreds of times before.

After the tube is in position she'll lie down, and during the next thirty or so minutes she will be asked and helped to turn from side to side. Her esophagus, stomach and duodenum will all be carefully examined. The ulcer will be located and photographed. Four tiny pieces will be taken from the edge of the crater and will be sent for microscopic examination. (She won't feel the biopsies at all; the stomach is not sensitive to that kind of procedure.) At the end of the examination, the instrument will be swiftly removed. Eloise, still a little drowsy, will be returned to her room.

Two days later the biopsy report will be available. In her case, no malignancy was found, and she will be kept on a diet and a schedule of antacids and sedatives in hopes of complete healing of her ulcer.

With the information gleaned from your history, combined with x-ray confirmation, acid secretory studies and examination by endoscopy, an accurate diagnosis is virtually assured. Rarely does an ulcer escape detection in more than a minuscule percentage of patients. If it is there, it will be found. And if it's not there, you will be reassured.

12

Medications for Ulcer

It is much easier to write upon a disease than upon a remedy. The former is in the hands of nature. . . . The latter will ever be subject to the whim, the inaccuracies and the blunders of mankind.

—William Withering (1741–1799)

Once a condition has been diagnosed as peptic ulcer, the two goals of therapy are to promote healing and prevent recurrence or flare-up. Since ulcer is a lifetime disease, it follows that the former is easier to accomplish than the latter.

The periodicity of ulcers makes it difficult to evaluate the effectiveness of any particular kind of treatment. Both gastric and duodenal ulcers undergo periods of flare-up and remission. Even without medical therapy an ulcer that has been activated and symptomatic for days, weeks, or months sometimes heals spontaneously, only to recur again after an indeterminate period of quiescence.

This phenomenon also helps to account for the many hundreds of ulcer remedies recommended over the years, that appear to be effective and are widely accepted before they are discovered to be of little or no use. Only controlled and randomly carried out trials determine what drugs or what sort of diet or other therapy actually affect the natural course of ulcers.

For example, in a recent British study, patients being prepared for planned surgery for duodenal ulcers were divided into two groups. One group was treated with a medication that effectively suppresses stomach-acid secretion, and the other with a placebo (sugar pill).* While four out of five of the people in the acid suppressant group reported complete healing of the ulcers in six weeks, one patient in every five in the placebo group was completely relieved of his or her symptoms, as was confirmed by x-ray and endoscopy. This study clearly demonstrates the effectiveness of the acid-suppressing drug. It also indicates that the ulcers of a significant number of people heal just as well with no treatment at all.

Nevertheless, based on the best evidence available to us at this time, certain regimens for the treatment of ulcers have survived the test of time and continue in widespread use today. While we now generally acknowledge that the causes of ulcers are complex and varied, all modern therapy is directed at suppression, neutralization or elimination of stomach acid.

ACID NEUTRALIZERS AND ANTACID THERAPY

There are a bewildering number of antacids, or acid-neutralizing agents, available for use. Few medications sold or

---

* Placebos have no known effect on any aspect of any disease. They are used to test for the possible psychological value of a drug.

produced by drug manufacturers have heavier advertising budgets than the antacids. This is a measure in part of the size of the market and the number of people using them.

The Functions of Antacids:

An antacid must first of all be safe, not only over the short term, but—particularly in a chronic disorder such as peptic ulcer—over long periods of time as well. One must also consider side effects. It should produce as few side effects as possible. Finally, an antacid should be effective. It should neutralize acid and in the process relieve pain. It also should encourage the ulcer to heal, and then help maintain it in a healed state. Unfortunately there is currently no antacid that fulfills these ideal requirements.

The two basic actions of antacids are the neutralization of acid by chemical reaction, and the physical absorption of it. Both sodium bicarbonate (simple baking soda) and calcium bicarbonate neutralize acid by combining with it to form another salt, water and carbon dioxide. About 1 gram of sodium or calcium bicarbonate (a teaspoon is about 5 grams) neutralizes approximately 200 cubic centimeters (a teacup holds about 240 cc.) of highly acid solution. As anyone who has ever relieved ulcer pain with baking soda can tell you, it is very effective, although it may cause some gassiness.

However, baking soda has some disadvantages. If it's taken in too large a dose or too frequently, it can cause the general body systems to become too alkaline. Furthermore, after the chemical reaction between baking soda and stomach acid is complete, stomach secretion may resume with increased vigor—the so-called rebound phenomenon.

Calcium carbonate is also a very efficient and effective antacid, but it can cause constipation. Also, overuse of calcium carbonate can lead to an abnormal rise in calcium levels in the blood and thus to a poisoning of the body systems. Paradoxically, elevation of blood calcium levels can also cause an *increased* acid secretion from the stomach. For these reasons calcium carbonate must be used with great caution. The combination of calcium carbonate and magnesium oxide (milk of magnesia) is a very useful medication; its use is limited, however, by the fact that diarrhea is a common side effect.

Aluminum hydroxide absorbs acid physically, although its major effect is chemical neutralization of acid. Aside from relatively mild constipation or diarrhea, the aluminum hydroxide medications don't have significant side effects. These aluminum-containing compounds enjoy the widest acceptability among people with ulcers, and also among physicians.

Antacids do not neutralize acid as efficiently in the tablet form as in the liquid. About one tablespoon of a liquid antacid is as effective as three tablets of the same antacid, although there is no doubt the tablet form is more convenient.

As any television addict can tell you, most of the antacids marketed today neutralize acid extremely well when mixed into a glass beaker full of it. Unfortunately, the stomach is not a glass beaker; not only does it secrete new acid all the time, but it's also emptying itself on a relatively continuous basis. These processes rapidly diminish the effect of antacid medications. Therefore, in the stomach the usual antacid acts for only twenty to forty minutes. This doesn't mean that pain won't be relieved for longer than that, only that the acid itself is buffered for just that length of time.

Do take your antacid at the right time. When the medication is taken an hour after a meal it's roughly twice as effective as a similar amount taken four hours after a meal. This is based on the fact that the stomach in a fasting state empties itself much more rapidly than one which has just been filled with a meal. Get into the habit of taking your medications accordingly.

Obviously, if there was a practical and acceptable way to completely eliminate or neutralize stomach acid, there would be no problem. This is not possible except under hospital conditions, with a twenty-four-hour-a-day flow of neutralizing substances through a tube in your stomach. No wonder there's so little agreement among physicians as to which antacid is best, and as to whether antacids do or do not have any effect at all on the natural course of ulcers.

There are many effective antacids on the market. In consultation with your physician and under careful supervision, experiment with two or three of the antacids he or she recommends to see which suits you the best. Obviously responses vary not only from person to person, but from time to time in the same person. If you're chronically constipated you may find the side effects of those effective antacids that cause looser stools actually beneficial. If you have the opposite problem, however, a constipating antacid may be more suitable.

NIGHT PAIN

No matter how well acid is neutralized during the day, either by food or by medication, once the stomach has emptied itself, acid secretions continue and may even rebound higher during the night. You obviously can't wake up every hour or even every few hours during the night to take an antacid or eat something. Some physicians advise a snack before bedtime; others claim that eating before bed only increases acid secretion later on during the night. While some have suggested taking antacids just before retiring, others have suggested keeping your antacid or a container of skim milk and cream on ice beside your bed to have on hand should you wake up.

My own advice is to experiment to determine what suits you best. Having a snack just before going to bed will keep some of you free of discomfort throughout the night. For others, a snack plus antacids may be best. For still others, milk and cream at the bedside may be most helpful. There is very little risk in such experimentation. The type of antacid you use and the schedule according to which you take it should be dictated by what relieves your symptoms and is relatively free of side effects. While your physician may have a favorite regimen and you should most certainly give it a try, both you and he are encouraged to modify it in an attempt to find out what works best for you.

The "Sippy" regimen, formulated just after the turn of the century, consists of taking antacids hourly in hopes of complete and continuous neutralization of stomach acid. This regimen requires hospitalization because it also includes emptying the stomach with a tube. It is not practical for the nonhospitalized patient.

ACID-SUPPRESSING DRUGS

The less acid your stomach produces, the easier it is to neutralize that which is present. In fact, any medication capable of just reducing the amount of acid to levels the neutralizers can cope with, or the normal protective mechanisms can defend against, would be very useful. This desire for a one-two punch on acid—first suppress its production as much as possible and then neutralize what is left over—has given rise to another class of medications somewhat less widely used than the acid neutralizers. As opposed to antacids, which neutralize either by chemically reacting with or by absorbing acid, the acid suppressors, or *anticholinergics,* act by reducing the amount of acid the stomach secretes. They do this by inhibiting the nervous impulses that directly stimulate both acid secretion and the release of the hormone gastrin.

Although the anticholinergics can be effective when taken in very large doses, stomach-acid secretion can't be suppressed completely by their use, and are mainly useful as adjuncts to the antacids. Unfortunately, the effect anticholinergics have on the body is not limited to the stomach. In fact, these drugs have a nerve-blocking effect throughout the body, and the functions of many organs besides the stomach can be interfered with. Anticholinergics depress the secretion of saliva and may cause your mouth to feel dry. They inhibit sweating and the secretions produced by the bronchial tubes. The pupils of the eyes dilate and vision blurs because the lenses lose some of their ability to accommodate to changes in distance. Acid suppressors usually increase one's heart rate. In the bladder, muscle tone and muscular contraction may be diminished or even wiped out by high doses, and people taking these medications may experience difficulty in emptying their bladders, a sometimes serious and disabling side effect.

But most importantly, at least in relation to our discussion of ulcers, the anticholinergic medications inhibit secretions from both the stomach and the pancreas. Unfortunately the stomach is somewhat less sensitive to these medications than are most of the other organs that are affected by them. Relatively large doses are needed to depress stomach-acid secretion, and the side effects from these doses often become unacceptable.

A time-honored medication for acid suppression, tincture of belladonna, derives its name, which means "beautiful lady," from the fact that Italian charmers enhanced the beauty and allure of their eyes by dilating their pupils with a drop or two. A group of medications resembling belladonna have been synthesized, and many of these have been manufactured and tested in hopes of developing one with a pinpoint effect on the stomach and fewer side effects. The evidence is poor, however, that this has been accomplished, and the consensus is that synthetic drugs have no particular advantages over the naturally produced belladonna.

In general these drugs are administered *until* the patient develops the side effects of blurred vision and dryness of the mouth. Indeed, my own professors in medical school used to advise us that the proper way to administer belladonna was to order a dose so large that *our own* eyes blurred! If you are especially dependent on sharpness of vision for your work, or if you intend to drive a car or perform some other function in which blurred vision would prove dangerous or inconvenient, you should take a dose of the medication that will fall just short of producing effects on your vision.

Belladonna does depress night-time acid secretion, hopefully allowing you to get a good night's rest free from symptoms attributable to the continuous production of acid. Many patients have reported excellent results with belladonna when used in this way, and if your doctor approves, I recommend that you try it. About the only advantage that the synthetic drugs may have over belladonna is a longer duration of action. Of course, this may be particularly desirable if night-time depression of acid is your goal.

Belladonna has also been used to reduce the acid secretion normally following a meal. To combat this secretion, you can take the medication from fifteen minutes to half an hour before you eat. Some important studies done by J. S. Fordtran and his coworkers at the University of Texas have shown that the acid-suppressing drugs work even in patients who have taken an acid-neutralizing medication following meals. The two drugs are possibly mutually supportive. Acid-reducing drugs decrease stomach tone and emptying just as they decrease bladder tone and emptying; in this way, they help keep the acid-neutralizing agent in the stomach somewhat longer.

You may develop an increased tolerance for belladonna, so after you have used it for a while it may be possible to increase the dose. *With your physician's approval and recommendations,* the dose may be readjusted in order to achieve the maximum effect on the stomach.

Finally, a word of warning. Patients whose stomachs are

partially obstructed due to scarring and distortion of the pyloric outlet (as a result of inflammation and healing of an ulcer) may find that *the relaxing effects of the acid-suppressing drugs increase the stomach's problems with emptying.* These drugs are therefore not useful for all classes of ulcer patients. If you are very elderly, have heart problems, eye trouble (glaucoma, for example) or bladder troubles, you are probably best advised not to use these medications at all.

Do these drugs aid in the healing of an ulcer, and do they help prevent its recurrence? Once again the problems of evaluating the effect of drug therapy on a disorder characterized, even without treatment, by remissions and flare-ups become apparent. Opinion seems to be fairly divided between those who think that these medications do in fact enhance healing and reduce recurrence and those who think there is no difference between groups who use the drug and those who do not. I myself don't believe they encourage ulcers to heal.

SEDATIVES

The role of stress and anxiety in the aggravation of an already existing ulcer has been examined at great length. A time-honored way to alleviate anxiety, restlessness and irritability is the use of sedatives. Unfortunately, sedatives also reduce your alertness. If you lead a relatively sedentary life or if you are going through a period when you don't need to make full use of your mental faculties—such as while you're on vacation or a holiday, or when your ulcer is in and of itself seriously interfering with your ability to function, or when you're hospitalized—sedation can prove to be helpful adjunctive therapy.

Sedatives may also be helpful in the control of night-time pain. *With your physician's approval,* they can be used in conjunction with antacids and anticholinergics and may help you get a good night's rest. Any of the so-called tranquilizers currently on the market or simply phenobarbital may be useful.

As you can see, the safe and efficient use of acid neutralizers (antacids), acid suppressors (anticholinergics) and sedatives is a complex business. These drugs are not suitable for self-medication. Consult with your doctor, and with him work out a regimen best suited to your individual needs. Although the discussion I have presented is somewhat detailed, my intention is to help you understand the way in which these medications work. I have not told you the brand names of any medications, nor the doses in which they are commonly prescribed. I do not intend for you to experiment with them by yourself. Please don't! The advantages of working with your physician to develop an effective program can be illustrated by Jacob's case.

HONOLULU, HAWAII. FEBRUARY 14, 1976

Jacob is a highly successful forty-two-year-old male Caucasian orchid grower with a thriving export business. His otherwise happy existence is marred by a chronic duodenal ulcer he has had for fifteen years. But Jake gets along rather well with his ulcer. It has never bled, the pain is controllable, and he has long periods of freedom from discomfort— sometimes up to six months.

When his ulcer flares up, Jake mobilizes all the tricks he and his doctor have worked out over the years. Jake cuts his smoking down to a half pack a day. He limits himself to one or two cups of coffee daily and eliminates alcohol altogether. He *never* takes any drug containing aspirin, so that's no problem. He restarts his bland diet and begins his antacid and anticholinergic regimen. At night he takes a snack, antacids and anticholinergics just before retiring. Night pain is only rarely a real problem for him.

Things weren't always so good for Jake and his ulcer. Much trial-and-error testing with a number of different antacids, acid suppressors and dietary restrictions was necessary before he and his doctor worked out an effective program. His physician would like Jake to maintain this program indefinitely, but it's not practical. Moreover, there's not much evidence that doing so will keep the ulcer from flaring up. So Jake does what he has to when he has to, and generally tries not to abuse his stomach between attacks. He knows that some things will cause trouble, and he avoids them.

Jake generally stays on his acute flare-up regimen for two to three weeks after the attack is over. Then, after consultation with his doctor, he resumes his normal life style.

13

Diet for People with Ulcers

Whatsoever was the father of a disease, an ill diet was the mother.

—Proverb

Our doctors . . . eat the melon and drink the new wine while they keep their patients tied down to syrups and slops.

—Michel de Montaigne (1533–1592)

For most of us a good meal is a basic element in the joy of living. The satisfaction derived from the warmth, sight, aroma and taste of good food is undeniable. The contentment that follows the alleviation of hunger pangs is a primal factor in well-being.

While most people believe that the gastrointestinal tract, particularly the stomach, is extremely sensitive, it is actually quite durable. Consider what effect the following treatment would have on the relatively thin epidermis of the inside of your forearm: Bathe this area with an irritating chemical mixed with very cold water. Fifteen minutes later repeat this treatment. Then rub the skin with a mixture of coarse grass, oil and some material roughly the consistency of dried sand. Pour a quarter of a pint of nearly boiling water on it, and then rub it again with a firm fibrous substance. Bathe the area again with a very hot liquid, and then with 90 proof alcohol. Although the extremes in thermal variation and even the coarseness of the material you ingest are modified somewhat by the process of chewing and swallowing (through the mouth, esophagus and stomach), this description, while exaggerated for the purposes of emphasis, represents approximately what happens to the gastrointestinal tract during the course of a meal: two Scotches on the rocks followed by a salad, a bowl of hot soup, the main course, some hot coffee or tea, and an after-dinner brandy or two.

Few aspects of treating people with ulcers have polarized physicians more than the subject of diet and its appropriate use. At one extreme are those who maintain that there is virtually no evidence showing that diet alters the natural course of the disorder. Patients should thus be allowed to eat whatever they desire as long as these foods do not cause discomfort. At the other extreme are the traditionalists, who believe that diet is important, if not fundamental, in treating ulcers. Moreover, patients *want* to be told what to eat.

> Now to perform a true physician's part,
> And show I am a perfect master of my art,
> I will prescribe what diet you should use,
> What food you ought to take, and what refuse.
> —Ovid (43 B.C.–A.D. 17?)

A number of fundamental questions should be considered even if well-documented answers are not yet available.

1. Can we identify specific foods that are important in the prevention of ulcer? Does *not* eating certain foods increase the incidence or retard the healing of ulcers?

2. Are there foods that cause or aggravate ulcers?

3. Do certain diets encourage the healing of ulcers or prevent their recurrence or relieve pain?

4. Does diet have a psychological value? Do patients eat some foods, or any foods, simply because it gives them oral gratification? Is this of value in managing ulcer?

5. Will patients follow diets during periods when they are between attacks as well as during an acute flare-up? Or are physicians merely prescribing diets because they believe it is expected of them?

6. Are self-selected diets, modified by what we know for certain to be harmful or of value, acceptable for people with ulcers?

7. Once the patient has been "cured" of an ulcer by surgical means, are there dietary factors that need to be considered so that both the possible side effects of surgery and the risk of "undoing" the cure can be minimized?

Deficient Diet as a Cause of Ulcers: Most people subconsciously associate the onset or continuation of ulcer discomfort with the foods they eat. However, perhaps it's not what they eat but what they don't eat that causes or aggravates ulcers. Direct and indirect evidence suggesting that malnutrition may or may not contribute to the development of ulcers has been reviewed in great detail in Chapter 7 (see especially pages 88–90), and will not be repeated here.

Throughout this book I have emphasized that overproduction of stomach acid is a final pathway to the development of ulcers. Studies show that vitamin B complex deprivation elevates both the volume and the concentration of acid juice secreted by the stomach. Vitamin C deficiency has also received a great deal of attention in ulcer research, since traditional ulcer diets consisting largely of dairy products, eggs and bland foods are notoriously poor in this vitamin. Levels of vitamin C in the blood of people with *untreated* ulcer drop markedly after therapy has been in effect for some time. People who treat themselves with milk, cream, cereals and eggs to the exclusion of vitamin C–containing foods may, after long periods of time, actually develop a scurvy-like syndrome.

Suffice it to say that while dietary deficiencies may be of considerable importance in causing ulcers, no firm conclusions concerning this can be drawn at this time. It doesn't seem possible to separate the effects of our diet from the effects of the rest of our environment. Although protein deficiency in particular and insufficient intake of vitamin A, B complex and C are often blamed for ulcers, there are no carefully controlled studies in humans corroborating this. However, a reasonably balanced diet of carbohydrates, fat, and protein is essential for well-being, and I strongly advocate such a diet for many reasons. I also recommend that you supplement your diet with polyvitamins if you are on a strict ulcer regimen.

FOODS AND BEVERAGES

A controversial topic of ulcer research is whether certain foods do or do not cause or aggravate ulcer. Most of the controversy seems to be based on opinion and "logic" rather than on evidence. For example, we know that acid is important in ulcer development, but this doesn't mean that "acid" foods or drinks (citrus juices, for example) are harmful. Ulcer patients often describe their pain as a burning sensation, but this doesn't necessarily mean that spicy or hot foods are harmful. There is no evidence for the assumption that the form, color, taste, consistency or smell of food has anything to do with its effect on the muscular or secretory activity of the stomach or its lining, or with the ultimate development of ulcers.

Caffeine and related agents *are* stomach-acid stimulants, and there is enough caffeine in moderate amounts of coffee, tea, chocolate and cola drinks to cause mildly increased acid production. But, except during an acute ulcer flare-up—at which time you should, if possible, completely eliminate them from your diet—they can be drunk in moderation. They may well aggravate an *active* ulcer, but the evidence that they cause ulcer or increase the frequency of attacks is weak and anecdotal, especially when they are consumed judiciously. Three to four cups of coffee or tea a day, or one or two cola drinks, and an occasional piece of chocolate should not cause problems. A paper published by the American Dietetic Association states that "spices, condiments, and highly seasoned foods are usually omitted on the basis that they irritate the gastric mucosa. However, experiments have indicated that no significant irritation occurs, even when most condiments are applied directly on the gastric mucosa. Exceptions are those items which *do* in fact cause gastric irritation, including black pepper, chili powder, caffeine, coffee, tea, cocoa, alcohol, and drugs." I know of no better way to express the current state of thinking on the matter.

Naturally, we are all sensitive to certain foods, but that doesn't mean that we either have an ulcer or are especially prone to developing one. Using a computerized questionnaire to determine sensitivity to certain foods, R. Earlam studied 100 people with x-ray-proven duodenal ulcers and 100 control people without ulcers. Here is a table from his informative study:

FOODS CAUSING INDIGESTION

Foods	Sensitive people with duodenal ulcer	Sensitive controls without ulcers
Pastry	77	4
Fried Food	72	9
Cucumber	62	16
Curry	57	5
Onions	54	10

Foods	Sensitive people with duodenal ulcer	Sensitive controls without ulcers
Pork	32	5
Fruit	31	1
Bacon	30	0
Beer	23	1
Cheese	18	1
Salads	18	1
Cake	16	1
Gravy	12	0
Lamb	12	1
Chocolate	11	0
Coffee	10	0
Tea	8	2

These important observations should be corroborated by other studies involving more subjects, but a number of useful conclusions can be drawn from this information. Certain foods *do* cause indigestion far more frequently in ulcer patients than in people who don't have ulcers, despite the lack of a satisfactory explanation for the phenomenon. These observations can act as a guide for you if you have an ulcer; you may want to modify the list based on your personal experience. Earlam's study shows that people have very individualized responses to certain foods. I find it especially interesting that the three foods least frequently reported as causing indigestion in the ulcer patients are chocolate, coffee and tea. Physicians especially should take note of this observation and modify their recommendations accordingly.

PSYCHOLOGY AND DIET

If, as many have suggested, patients with duodenal ulcer require an inordinate amount of oral gratification to pacify their conflicts and anxieties, then eating could certainly be expected to be one of the most socially acceptable and prevalent ways of satisfying these needs.

Wolowitz, a psychologist, and Wagonfeld, a psychiatrist, have tested Alexander's psychoanalytic hypothesis that oral passive (sucking) wishes, as opposed to oral aggressive (biting) wishes, play an important role in peptic ulcer. They studied thirty-eight patients with peptic ulcer and sixty-two with other diagnoses. Unfortunately, they did not differentiate between patients with duodenal ulcers and those with gastric ones. They rated their study group on the basis of preferences among 103 food items listed on a questionnaire; some choices were considered to be oral aggressive and some oral passive.

The ulcer patients picked 58.1 percent of the oral passive choices, while the patients without ulcers chose 50.1 percent, an 8 percent difference between the two groups. On that slim, though "statistically significant" margin, Wolowitz and Wagonfeld based the following conclusion: "As *predicted* [emphasis mine], the ulcer group's [average] oral passive score was significantly higher than the non-ulcer group, thereby supporting Alexander's contention that all passive psychological needs play an important role in the etiology of peptic ulcer."

This is an oversimplification of a very complex phenomenon; as a generalization it has serious problems. One would expect a group of oral-dependent people to eat more often and to consume greater amounts of food than a control group. In fact, there isn't much evidence that patients "feed their ulcers." Ulcer patients on the whole tend to weigh about the same or slightly less than comparable groups of people without ulcers. Then too, if food is gratification, eating should relieve ulcer symptoms in a very high percentage of cases. It is commonly believed that food relieves the symptoms of ulcer. In the study previously mentioned, Earlam noted that the pain of ulcers was essentially unaffected by diet and was *not* related to meals. Although the largest portion of the patients reported that their symptoms were most intense just before a meal, 40 percent said food made the pain worse! Seventeen patients thought their weight increased because of indigestion, but forty-five thought it decreased and thirty-six said it was unchanged. Seventy of the hundred patients did believe that they ate more because of the pain, and the fact that very few of them gained weight is possibly related to other unidentified factors.

The evidence for Alexander's hypothesis that oral dependence is a critical factor in ulcer development must stand on its own merits. While I don't subscribe to this theory, I'd like to reserve judgment until more scientifically controlled and statistically valid proof is available.

DIET AS MEDICAL THERAPY FOR ULCER

In 1911, the same year that Marie Curie won the Nobel Prize for the discovery of radium, a physician by the name of B. W. Sippy introduced a regimen that was to have a profound and enduring effect on the treatment of ulcers by diet. His program, still used today in many clinics throughout the world, consists of alternating milk and alkali on an hourly basis *during the acute phase of an ulcer flare-up.* For now, though, I would like to discuss dietary factors of importance in the *long-term therapy* of people with ulcers and in *the periods between attacks,* some of which may last many months or years.

In the literature on the value of diet in managing ulcer you will find everything from elaborate hour-by-hour recommendations and detailed outlines to the attitude that "there is no evidence that diet affects either the causation of ulcer, the incidence of complications, the length of time it takes to heal an ulcer, or the duration of time between recurrences." Somewhere lies a middle ground that I'd like to explore with you. While scientific proof that diet is beneficial in ulcer disease has not been forthcoming, dietary considerations are important if for no other reason than that many people *think* they are.

Several basic principles should be taken into consideration in determining what type of diet the person with an ulcer should adhere to. At the very minimum your diet should provide you with enough calories so that you don't lose or gain a lot of weight. Also, it should not contain foods that cause you to have pain.

The rationale for a bland diet is weak and poorly supported by the available scientific evidence. In fact, there is virtually no evidence that milk or milk products and bland diets reduce gastric acidity. As J. S. Fordtran, one of the most authoritative figures in the field, has stated, hourly milk and cream intake tends to maintain acid concentration in the stomach at a high level. Fordtran has concluded that no change in the clinical course of peptic ulcer can be attributed to the use of a bland diet or to the elimination of juices, and that there is no convincing evidence that any specific diet will be associated with less gastric acidity than a normal diet of your own choosing.

Milk does relieve duodenal ulcer pain, although its acid-neutralizing effect is minimal. Its buffering action, however, could conceivably be outweighed by its ability to stimulate acid production. In fact, most foods tend to increase acid secretion to some extent. Although protein, for example, provides the greatest buffering action, it's also the most powerful stimulus to acid secretion. While the benefits of milk in ulcer diets is still widely debated, it has been used less and less over the past twenty years, and strict insistence on it during periods when you are free from ulcer pain doesn't make much sense.

The American Dietetic Association, Fordtran, and others have also concluded that provided they are well-chewed and mixed with saliva, roughage or coarse foods (for example, fruit skins, lettuce, nuts and celery) have no adverse affect on duodenal ulcers. Only if your teeth are in poor condition should the grinding of foods or the eating of a puréed diet be necessary.

Fordtran and many others, including me, have concluded, based on a number of reliable investigations, that there *is* some value in frequent small feedings in people suffering a flare-up of duodenal ulcer. Frequent small feedings during an ulcer attack seem to lower acid and are preferred. H. M. Spiro, a prominent gastroenterologist at Yale, makes the following points: An ordinary meal is known to neutralize gastric content for about one-half to one hour, but is then followed by increased acid secretion. In a study by Lennard-Jones comparing the effects on the stomach of two different bland diets with that of a normal British meal, *neither* lowered stomach acid. In fact, the normal diet was associated with lower acid. The more frequent the feedings, however, the lower the acid level observed. A meal given every two hours is thus preferable to one given every four hours.

UNDERSTANDING AND WILLINGNESS TO FOLLOW A DIET

While people with ulcers wish to understand their disorder and strongly desire to do whatever is reasonable to control it, confusion concerning the best diet for ulcer patients to follow is widespread. In a 1967 article, H. P. Roth and H. S. Caron reported on the misconceptions patients often have concerning the diets that have been recommended to them. In a thoughtful and provocative study, they interviewed one hundred and fifty-two men with ulcers and thirty of their wives.

These patients didn't doubt that diet was potentially important in the control of their ulcers. Many described a "good" diet as one which corresponded well with the so-called Sippy regimen of hourly milk and alkali, which doctors generally reserve for periods when ulcers flare up. But many of the patients believed that this program was to be followed for life, a course of action which would "lead to a more strict and comprehensive diet than that intended . . . [and] would be difficult if not impossible to follow."

Even more importantly, however, the subjects didn't really understand that foods which *stimulate* acid should be restricted, rather than those which *seem* acid, or which they believed were irritating to the stomach. The authors concluded that patients were ignoring the recommended diets and were employing "a simple test based on symptoms, that is, a food may be eaten if it does not produce symptoms."

Physicians and people with ulcers alike must understand the subtle rationale for dietary management of ulcers. Foods and beverages that seem acid (such as citrus juices) don't necessarily cause an increase in acid secretion. They are often less acid than stomach juice and by mixing with it actually lower the overall acid content.*

DIET FOR THE ACUTE FLARE-UP OF ULCER

When an ulcer is acutely activated, a much more rigorous approach to diet is required. People who know they have a duodenal ulcer, or who think they do, should be under a physician's care. This is particularly important if you have an ulcer and are suffering from a flare-up. *Neglect or in-*

---

* Fordtran has stated that the data on citrus juices is somewhat confused, and a final judgment cannot be made at this time. If such juices *do* cause increased acidity, he feels, it is probably due to stimulation of acid secretion or to reduction of the buffering effect of a mixed meal, rather than to their relative acidity to start with. Haggard and Greenberg report that within ninety minutes after a meal during which pineapple, grape, orange, and grapefruit juices were evaluated, all of these juices except grapefruit were associated with *less acidity than when plain water was taken.*

difference on your part concerning this phase of the natural course of ulcer disease can lead to disaster. The complications of obstruction, perforation and bleeding are much too serious to be self-treated. Although a patient suffering from acute activity of an ulcer can sometimes be successfully managed on an outpatient or ambulatory basis, many of you will have to stay home or be hospitalized.

Here are a few basic principles in the proper management of the acute attack.

1. You must obtain your physician's advice and follow his recommendations.

2. It may be advisable to restrict you to your home or to have you briefly hospitalized.

3. The Sippy regimen is probably most appropriate during this phase. It consists of taking hourly or half-hourly doses of skim milk and acid-neutralizing medications. The regimen can be supplemented by acid-suppressing agents.

4. If there is any role for a bland diet in the management of ulcer, it is during the acute attack. A typical bland diet, kindly provided by the Twin City Dietary Association, can be found on the opposite page. It is written in accordance with the American Dietetic Association Position Paper of 1971: "This diet omits only those foods sufficiently supported by scientific evidence to cause gastric irritation. Individual diets may need to be adjusted considering specific food intolerances."

5. Coffee, tea, chocolate, cocoa, cola drinks, alcohol, and aspirin *must* be completely eliminated. While some of these can be taken in moderation between attacks, aspirin in particular should never be taken by patients with ulcer.

6. Bed rest often contributes to the relief of duodenal ulcer symptoms and may be desirable. But there is no evidence that holidays or vacations are especially beneficial during the acute attack.

7. Mild sedatives are also of value in treating the patient whose ulcer has flared up.

8. Except for short periods of time these regimens are far

BLAND DIET

GUIDELINES:
1. Eat small quantities of food at regular intervals.
2. Eat slowly.
3. If a food causes distress, eliminate it for a period of time.

To provide essential nutrients, include each day a minimum of:

2 servings of milk or milk products
4 servings of bread or cereal products
4 servings of fruits and vegetables
2 servings of meat or a substitute

Desserts, fats, sweets and other foods in moderation will add variety, energy and flavor.

FOOD:	OMITTED:
Beverage	Coffee, tea, colas, chocolate, cocoa and alcoholic beverages
Breads	Any containing chocolate or cocoa
Cereal	Any containing chocolate or cocoa
Desserts	Any containing chocolate or cocoa
Fats	Salad dressings prepared with omitted spices
Fruits	None
Meat or Substitute	Any prepared with omitted spices
Potato or Substitute	Any prepared with omitted spices
Soup	Any prepared with omitted spices
Sweets	Any containing chocolate or cocoa
Vegetables	Any prepared with omitted spices
Miscellaneous	Black pepper, white pepper, chili powder, cayenne, curry powder, red pepper

too restrictive for normal life. If after a few days to a week complete or virtually complete relief from symptoms has not occurred, serious consideration should be given to surgery.

9. After symptoms have been controlled, and evidence of ulcer healing has been established, the regimen may be slowly modified by resumption of a more normal and palat-

able diet. Drinking beverages known to increase gastric secretion should only be embarked upon very slowly. If they can be eliminated altogether, this would be best. If this isn't possible, I would prefer they be taken only in moderation.

CAN DIETS UNDO THE CURE EFFECTED BY SURGERY?

Chapter 15 discusses some of the special problems you may encounter after an operation for cure of your ulcer. In general, though, provided your diet is nutritious and doesn't cause obesity or malnutrition, you may eat anything that doesn't bother you. Some things you were able to eat before surgery may have to be restricted, but more likely many things you couldn't eat before will then be easily tolerated. Experiment and enjoy!

14

Surgery for Peptic Ulcers

Surgeons must be very careful
When they take the knife!
Underneath their fine incisions
Stirs the culprit, Life.
                    —Emily Dickinson

For many, just a mention of the operating room conjures up visions of a chamber of horrors. But while only a relatively small number of people with ulcers require surgery, you should recognize that the modern operating room and the purposes for which it is intended represent the culmination of civilization's best efforts. For those who love it, need it, or can benefit from it, it is a sanctuary.

It can be the most peaceful, controlled, receptive environment imaginable. It is clean; it is quiet. It is bright where it should be and muted where appropriate. It is climatically unobtrusive and it is protected. Seven or more people devote their entire physical, emotional and intellectual efforts to the care of the person alseep under the sheets. Surgeons know that they can stand in one square foot for two, ten or more hours, without fatigue, without the need to empty the bladder, and without the intrusion of unrelated thoughts. Only when one leaves the amphitheater do the messages, phone calls, obligations and responsibilities of the real world descend. The contrast only serves to emphasize the tranquillity of the environment just left.

The operating room is also a theater, with a stage, actors, a director, props and prop-people, spotlights, costumes, scripts, and often an audience. It is unreal. It is *sur*real.

In an age when men walk the moon and machines circle the planets, it's hard to believe that the first successful operation for removal of part of the stomach was performed less than one hundred years ago. In 1881, fourteen years before Roentgen discovered the x-ray and seventy-five years after telescopic examination of the stomach was first attempted, a forty-four-year-old woman presented herself to Billroth, the father of abdominal surgery, for removal of a cancer at the lower end of her stomach. This was carried out in the famous hospital at the University of Vienna, Allgemeines Krankenhaus. One can only imagine the excitement caused by Billroth's triumph. Three years later, Rydygier of Poland performed the first successful operation for the treatment of peptic ulcer. These were the first steps in the evolution of modern surgery for diseases of the stomach.

In the late nineteenth century the processes of digestion were poorly understood. Only rudimentary appreciation of the underlying causes of ulcers existed. Surgical techniques were primitive, and surgical instruments unsophisticated. Blood transfusion, although first attempted in the seventeenth century, was uncommon and unsafe. Consistently reliable anesthesia was still many years in the future, although ether had been in use since 1842. The intravenous injection of drugs and fluid was still in its very early stages. Understanding of the causes of infection was just beginning to spread and be accepted. Rubber surgical gloves were not used in America until the winter of 1890. Caps and masks were not worn in the operating theaters; refined suture material did not exist. An understanding of ulcers and of the principles which govern safe, modern surgery developed and spread only very slowly. Still, by the middle of the twentieth century, the digestive process was better understood, and the ideas basic to a comprehension of ulcer disease were established.

While precise figures are not available, an estimated 10 to 20 million Americans suffer from ulcers. But only a fraction undergo ulcer surgery each year. Obviously ulcers in the vast majority of the people who have them can be more or less satisfactorily managed by nonsurgical means. However, while medical treatment can *control* peptic ulcer, surgery *cures* it. I've heard my children say that "a sweater is something you wear when your mother is cold." It has been my feeling that surgery for ulcers is all too often something you have when your *doctor* can no longer stand the pain. *His* fear, anxieties and prejudices should not override your need or desire for definitive surgical treatment.

Not every person with peptic ulcer can benefit from surgery. For some, the disease is so mild that it can easily be controlled or at least tolerated with relatively minor medical treatment. For others, the risk of operation may be so great as to outweigh the potential rewards. Only one out of seven or eight people with ulcers ultimately has surgery, and there are some very specific reasons why one particular patient is operated on and another isn't. For many of you, surgery is simply not recommended. Some people refuse to undergo surgery. But for others, there may be no choice.

ELECTIVE VERSUS EMERGENCY SURGERY

Unfortunately there is no really convenient time to have surgery. I have never known a single person who looked forward with enthusiasm to an operation. There are children to make arrangements for, business trips to be postponed, exams and classes to be made up, and so forth. At best, surgery is an imposition, an intrusion on the normal routines of life. At worst, it can be frightening and even terrifying. Only a fool or an incompetent, or the desperately uncomfortable, think of surgery as an attractive alternative to the status quo. People commonly resent and fear the need for surgery to control their peptic ulcers. It sometimes seems almost a reproach. "Why," they ask, "does it have to be?"

Modern surgery in competent hands is extremely safe and effective. Under planned circumstances, when you are properly prepared and your general physical condition is brought up to the optimum level, the risk to life is less than one in a hundred. In the experience of many of us, it is more like one in two hundred.

If surgery must be performed on an emergency basis, when you are suffering from a life-threatening complication or when you are not in top physical shape, the risk to life soars. It can be as high as 20 to 40 percent. Obviously, therefore, surgery is best performed *before* the circumstances become urgent and pressing. When one considers the safety and success of an *elective* operation, performed when you are in relatively good health, it seems absurd that surgery is deferred for as long as it sometimes is.

REASONS FOR OPERATING

The Intractable Ulcer: By far the most common cause of ulcer surgery, the intractable ulcer is the only ulcer condition permitting a voluntary operation scheduled at the convenience of both the patient and the surgeon. The term "intractable" simply means that the ulcer cannot be satisfactorily managed by medication. But, as these case histories of patients with intractable ulcer can illustrate, what appears to be satisfactory control for one patient may not be for another.

SCARSDALE, NEW YORK. OCTOBER 5, 1973

Benjamin is a hard-working highly successful fifty-eight-year-old optometrist. His first ulcer symptoms appeared in 1943 shortly after he was inducted into the Army. For nine years the symptoms consisted only of pain, which was moderately well controlled with medication. But in 1952 and again in 1963 Benjamin's ulcer hemorrhaged and he had to be hospitalized. In both instances, the bleeding was well controlled by medication, so no blood transfusions were required.

Benjamin continued to have intermittent flare-ups of ulcer symptoms. Over the course of years he lost an average of three to five days of work each spring and each autumn due to incapacitation by pain. Although he's a gourmet cook and connoisseur of wines, he can't indulge his tastes very often, for whenever he does, his ulcer flares up.

His brother, a prominent Philadelphia gastroenterologist, has repeatedly warned him not to consider surgery. By 1973, however, he has had it with his ulcer; he's mentally prepared for and demands permanent relief. During the period before his operation he will be carefully reevaluated and prepared so that surgery will be as safe as possible.

This case study provides us with a typical example of a person with an intractable ulcer. Despite intelligent and conscientious medical therapy, he'd had two episodes of bleeding, neither of which was sufficiently compelling to require emergency surgery. However, thirty years of intermittent symptoms had deprived him of much of the joy of life. Even though he has had long periods of freedom from complaints, the constant threats of flare-up finally brought him to the decision to undergo surgery.

Ben had his operation and has been completely free of symptoms for four years. His only complaint, he reports with some amusement, is that he sometimes misses the gnawing pain in his belly. Thirty years of symptoms will do that.

Helen is a forty-seven-year-old extremely competent executive secretary to the president of a major corporation. She first developed ulcer symptoms in 1946, while she was working for a very overbearing and demanding boss. Her father also died that same year.

She's had intermittent symptoms for over twenty-five years, largely consisting of pain. Occasionally during particularly severe and prolonged episodes of flare-up, she notes that her abdomen is distended; during these periods she has sometimes felt nauseated or has thrown up. However, intensive medication programs have always managed to relieve her symptoms. Sometimes she has enjoyed long periods of freedom from complaints.

Recently, however, the attacks have become more frequent and more prolonged. Medication does not bring the relief it used to. Although she has lost no time from work, her efficiency has dropped. She is depressed, uncomfortable and fatigued by her condition. Surgery has been recommended by her physician, and within two weeks she will enter the hospital to be operated on.

Helen, too, had an intractable ulcer. She had never bled and had been able to perform satisfactorily in a very demanding job. She'd had only occasional symptoms of incomplete obstruction of the stomach outlet. She could perhaps have gone on virtually indefinitely as she was. However, when her physician advised surgery, she weighed the pros and cons carefully and sought the opinion of another physician. He concurred, and she opted for an operation.

She underwent surgery and has done very well for the past two years. She's not, however, completely free of symptoms. Rich desserts, thick soups, milkshakes and meals heavy in carbohydrates cause her to break out in sweat, her heart to pound and her head to feel light. She has learned to avoid these foods. She feels that she's been well compensated for their loss by the many things she can now eat that used to cause her discomfort, and by her otherwise complete freedom from symptoms.

The subjectivity of the term "intractable" makes it almost impossible to define except in terms of your personal needs and requirements. Whether or not to operate is basically a matter for you and your physician to decide. Together you will determine the exact moment when an ulcer has become intractable.

In a recently published monograph for surgeons on "A Physiologic Approach to the Surgical Management for Duodenal Ulcer," I made the following statement:

> In general, the patient . . . who despite prolonged and reasonably well-controlled non-operative management continues to be exposed to a significant health hazard as a result of the disease, or who can no longer function satisfactorily because of it, is considered intractable. Frequent small hemorrhages, chronic in nature and not sufficiently severe at any one time to require transfusion; recurrent episodes of stomach obstruction transiently alleviated by medical therapy; nutritional disability either in terms of semi-starvation, or obesity as a result of a high-caloric ulcer diet; and the inability to maintain a *reasonable quality of life,* all contribute to the picture of intractability.

The Bleeding Duodenal Ulcer: Some people must have an emergency operation because of life-threatening complications. The most common and compelling of these is bleeding from the ulcer. Bleeding is the number one cause of mortality from the disorder, and almost half the patients who die from ulcers do so from bleeding.

Roughly 2 percent of people with ulcers will have some bleeding from their ulcers some time during the course of their disease. While about one person in seven experiences hemorrhage as the very first sign of ulcers, most people admitted to the hospital for bleeding ulcers are suffering from a second, third or fourth attack. Since the longer an ulcer is present the more likely it is to bleed, most bleeding ulcers have been present for some time. As the ulcer penetrates the wall of the duodenum or of the stomach, the juices may digest a hole in a major blood vessel. The result can be minor bleeding, or it can be uncontrollable hemorrhage. David is typical of patients with a bleeding duodenal ulcer.

SALT LAKE CITY, UTAH. FEBRUARY 24, 1975

David is a fifty-two-year-old white male insurance agent. He's had a duodenal ulcer. Until recently his symptoms consisted largely of pain in the upper middle part of his abdomen just below the central portion of the breastbone, but now the pain also penetrates through to his back. He's already had three episodes of bleeding from his ulcer—one in 1954, one in 1967, and one in 1969. The first two didn't require blood transfusions, but in 1969 he had to have three pints of blood before the hemorrhage could be brought under control. Surgery was advised at that time, but he declined.

Just recently, David has passed two large black tarry bowel movements. He immediately recognized the significance of these and reported to the emergency room at the university hospital. His physician met him there and promptly admitted him to the hospital. Although his blood pressure was normal, his pulse rate was 120 beats per minute. Blood testing showed that his hemoglobin was 40 percent below normal.

During his physical examination, he vomited half a pint of bright red blood. Transfusion was begun immediately, and he was taken to an examining room, where endoscopic examination of his stomach and duodenum revealed that his old ulcer was bleeding. Over the next day he was given five more units of blood and intensive medical therapy was begun, but he continued to pass bloody bowel movements and to show persistent evidence of bleeding from the ulcer.

Despite blood replacement his hemoglobin remained at 40 percent below normal. Surgery was urgently recommended and accepted by both David and his family. He was operated upon and his ulcer oversewn. The vagus nerves to his stomach were cut and the pyloric outlet enlarged. He recovered and was discharged from the hospital in nine days.

David did well following his surgery for bleeding duodenal ulcer. He survived an operation for an extremely serious and dangerous complication. Others with massively bleeding ulcers are not so fortunate.

The Perforated Duodenal Ulcer: When the defenses that normally protect the membranes lining your stomach wall or duodenum are overwhelmed by the corrosive action of digestive juice, the tissue becomes eroded. The inflammation gradually penetrates through the layers of the wall, and eventually (if the process continues unchecked) complete through-and-through penetration will take place. In gastric ulcers the perforation may occur on the lesser curvature or on the front wall, allowing passage of stomach juices and food directly into the peritoneal cavity and giving rise to peritonitis. In the case of the perforating duodenal ulcer, if the ulcer is on the back wall, it may penetrate into the pancreas, an organ that lies behind the duodenum, or into a major artery located in that same general area. If the ulcer is on the front surface of the duodenum, perforation may allow the stomach's contents to pour freely into the abdominal cavity.

Why ulcers finally perforate is not known. However, a number of possibilities exist. The following ditty from a charming book written by Sir Zachary Cope offers some ideas on the subject:

> The reasons why they rupture are more clear—
> A slight increase of pressure would appear
> Sufficient to make ulcer's thinned-out base
> Give way so that the gastric contents race

Like waterfall into coelomic space.
A satisfying meal, a sudden fall—
A trivial strain, or nothing much at all,
May precede perforation—yes and it's
Curious how many ruptured in the Blitz.*

In contrast to the bleeding duodenal ulcer, the freely perforating ulcer is likely to occur earlier in the development of the disease. The development of a perforated ulcer is usually a rather sudden and frightening experience. Richard is a case in point.

CAMP PENDLETON, CALIFORNIA. JULY 15, 1974

Richard is a twenty-year-old white high school graduate. He recently joined the Marine Corps. Born and brought up in Boise, Idaho, until his arrival in southern California he had never been more than 150 miles from his home. Sullen, hostile, aggressive and anxious, he's made no friends in the service and is regarded by both his superiors and his fellow trainees as a troublemaker. Except for occasional hunger pains and "indigestion," he has had no recognizable illnesses.

Richard's basic training has been going badly; for six weeks he's been more or less continuously in trouble. The military food disagrees with him, and he's had an "upset stomach" intermittently almost since the day he arrived.

Within two hours of a particularly abusive tongue-lashing by the corporal in command of his platoon, he's hit by a sudden breathtakingly severe abdominal pain. His "belly feels like it's on fire." He lies doubled up on his cot. When his sergeant finds him there, he is immediately sent to the emergency room at the camp hospital.

The diagnosis of perforated ulcer is made on the basis of the sudden onset of pain, his rigid abdomen, and x-rays,

---

* The reference to the blitz, incidentally, is of some passing interest. During the heavy bombing raids on London during World War II the incidence of perforated peptic ulcer skyrocketed. See Chapter 7 for a more detailed comment on this phenomenon.

which show free air in his abdominal cavity. Within ninety minutes he is taken to the operating room.

The mortality rate for patients with a perforated duodenal ulcer is not as high as the rate for those with uncontrolled bleeding ulcer. Perforated gastric ulcer is more life-threatening than perforated duodenal ulcer, but it too is relatively less dangerous than bleeding ulcers.

Although a nonsurgical treatment for perforated ulcers has been described, almost all of them are treated immediately by surgery. Surgery is successful in most cases, but success and survival depend on many factors, one of which is your age. Survival also depends on your general physical condition, what kind of material has been spilled into your abdominal cavity, and the length of time between the perforation and the treatment by surgery. The overall mortality for perforated ulcers is about 12 to 15 percent no matter how they are treated, although it can be much higher or lower depending on the factors just mentioned. Perforation is therefore a very serious complication.

Depending on the operation performed, the patient can be completely cured or (in about 70 percent of cases) can continue to have ulcer symptoms. Half of those who still have symptoms will ultimately require more definitive surgery. This is usually carried out on planned rather than emergency elective basis. In Richard's case a so-called definitive operation was carried out at the time of the emergency surgery. His ulcer was cured, and he had no further stomach complaints.

The Obstructed Duodenal Ulcer: The fourth complication that may require surgery is blockage of the pyloric outlet of the stomach. This can occur as a result of inflammation, swelling and distortion by scar.

Most pyloric-outlet obstructions occur as a result of long-standing duodenal ulcer, but occasionally a low-lying stomach ulcer can also cause obstruction. Repeated bouts of inflammation and healing lay down scar tissue in the area, thicken the wall and distort the passage. Ultimately the passage may be completely stopped up. The blockage usually takes years to evolve. Harry's story is an example.

MINNEAPOLIS, MINNESOTA. JANUARY 28, 1977

A sixty-nine-year-old white male World War II veteran, Harry has been a farmer and part-time carpenter for most of his adult life. He has a moderately good work record, but he's a hard drinker and a heavy smoker, and has been for forty-five years. His first ulcer symptoms appeared back in 1949; since his discharge from the Army, he has been admitted some twenty-seven times to various Veterans Administration hospitals. Most of these admissions have been for pain, although several of them have been for small episodes of hemorrhage and the last three were for intermittent bouts of nausea and vomiting. Over the past eighteen months he has lost thirty pounds. He's been offered surgery many times but has either refused it or has left the hospital against his doctor's advice.

He has now been admitted to the Minneapolis VA hospital for vomiting of seventy-two hours' duration and an inability to hold down food or liquids. X-ray examination reveals that the outlet from his stomach is completely obstructed; endoscopic examination confirms the diagnosis.

Harry was placed on suction by a tube passed into his stomach through his nostril, but this time the stoppage doesn't appear to be giving way to medical therapy. Surgery is therefore urgent, and three days later Harry will be operated upon. The period between his admission and the operation will be used to correct the loss of body fluids and to restore body salts lost because of the vomiting, as well as to improve his lung function, which smoking has diminished.

As in this case, sometimes the process occurs sufficiently slowly so that the patient is forewarned. Mild episodes of abdominal bloating, occasionally accompanied by vomiting, may occur. They may be relieved by a liquid diet plus medication, and often occur at intervals over several months or more. Although partial or complete blockage is usually not considered an emergency, prolonged delay in surgical treatment should be avoided; in most instances an operation is ultimately required.

Most operations designed to handle obstructed ulcers are the same ones used for intractable ulcers. Obstruction can also occur in conjunction with bleeding, but this does not change the kind of operation used to correct the problem. Properly performed, the operation has the desired effect in a very high percentage of patients, and surgery for obstruction is much safer and better tolerated than is emergency surgery for bleeding or for perforation. In this case, Harry did fine and has returned to work.

PROPHYLACTIC SURGERY FOR PREVENTION OF COMPLICATIONS

An additional but relatively uncommon reason for surgery in people with ulcers comes up when a person is about to undergo an operation for an unrelated disorder. In order to prevent a flare-up or complication of the ulcer during the postoperative period, which may develop from the stress of the primary operation, the surgeon may perform a curative prophylactic ulcer operation at the same time.

A prophylactic ulcer operation may be added to operations for the treatment of such conditions as abdominal aortic aneurysm (arteriosclerotic weakening and ballooning of the major vessel from the heart), gallbladder disease, hiatus hernia, liver and pancreatic disorders requiring surgery, tumors of the abdominal organs, and kidney transplantations.

MODERN SURGERY FOR PEPTIC ULCER

Although more than fifty kinds of operations have been advocated in the treatment of peptic ulcer since Rydygier's first success in 1884, it's not surprising that only a few are still in current use. Some have proven ineffective. Some are too dangerous. In some the side effects and aftermaths are intolerable, worse than the conditions they were devised to relieve. Through trial and error and careful evaluation of results in thousands of patients over long periods of time, and as a result of a better understanding of the processes leading to ulcers, surgeons have developed at least three operations that are safe, effective and well-tolerated.

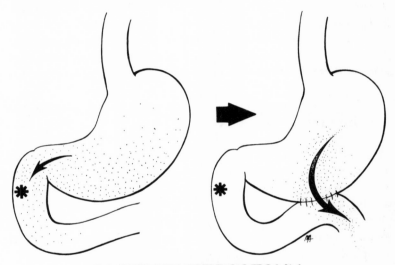

GASTROENTEROSTOMY:
Re-routing of acid stomach juices before they bathe an ulcer.

The painfully slow evolution of these achievements was due in large measure to lack of appreciation of the true nature of the cause of ulcers. Following the demonstration by Billroth that part of the stomach could be surgically removed and the patient could survive, and Rydygier's first successful operation for an ulcer, German and Austrian surgeons advocated and performed a flurry of operations.

The initial operative procedures were based on the rather naive idea that simply shielding the ulcer from acid could effect permanent cure in a large percentage of patients. Surgery was therefore used to reroute gastric juice directly from the stomach to the small bowel (gastroenterostomy), bypassing the stomach and its ulcer (see Figure 3). The idea was not entirely without merit and many ulcers responded by healing. However, to the dismay of all concerned, while the patient's old ulcer healed, new ulcers often appeared in the small bowel where the gastric juice now bathed the unprotected intestinal lining.

In retrospect, it is clear that the three fundamental concepts on which safe and curative surgery for ulcers are based were not yet fully understood at the turn of the century. These principles are:

1. In the duodenal ulcer patient, activated stomach juice can overwhelm normal defense mechanisms. In the gastric ulcer patient, relatively normal volumes of acid gastric juice appear to be too much for the existing defenses.

2. While many factors contribute to the development of peptic ulcer, the relative overproduction of acid is the underlying cause. Thus the control of acid secretion represents a direct approach to the control of ulcer and serves as a basis for all modern medical and surgical therapy.

3. The three most important factors in the production or overproduction of acid are (1) the stimuli that arise in the central nervous system and that are carried to the stomach by way of the vagus nerves; (2) the hormone gastrin, which is liberated from the antrum, the lower portion of the stomach; and (3) the number and sensitivity of the stomach's cells that respond to these stimuli by making the acid. These are the key elements in the control of acid.

Successful control of ulcer depends on reduction or neutralization of acid. It isn't necessary to completely eliminate acid, but simply to suppress it, at least to levels at which the protective mechanisms of the gastrointestinal tract can handle it and prevent self-digestion. This can be accomplished in one of three ways: reduce stimuli to the oversecreting stomach; significantly reduce the actual amount of tissue that secretes acid (reduction in the stomach's cell mass); or enhance the inhibitory mechanisms that normally regulate stomach-acid secretion.

Unfortunately, only the first two are possible with currently available means. Therefore, modern surgery for peptic ulcer depends on an assault on the stimuli to gastric secretion and/or the reduction of acid-secreting tissue. Even early in the development of this field it was appreciated that the ulcer itself, particularly when it is in the duodenum, does not necessarily have to be removed. It will heal if acid is sufficiently reduced. The poor results obtained with operations that simply rerouted acid stomach juices led to the search for more effective and safer operations. Of the many which have evolved, only three (really two) are extensively used today.

I. Sub-total Gastrectomy: Actual surgical removal of two-thirds to three-quarters of the lower portion of the stomach was the first operation that proved to effectively control ulcers (see Figure 4). In 1911 a German by the name of Polya, laboring under the misconception that the antrum is capable of secreting acid, recommended that this part of the stomach, plus a little more, be removed. This constituted a landmark modification of previously recommended operations, and it rapidly replaced the simple rerouting of stomach juices favored in the Austrian and German clinics.

In the 1920's the technique was brought to the United States by Lewisohn and Berg in New York and by Strauss in Chicago. American surgeons initially greeted the operation with derision and misgivings. During an early presentation of the idea at a major medical meeting, an irate surgeon interrupted the speaker by stating, "If someone wanted to cut out my *good stomach* to cure an ulcer in my *sick duodenum,* I would run faster than he"—and the audience cheered.

Nevertheless, the operation rapidly gained acceptance and for more than thirty-five years was the most commonly performed throughout the world. Hundreds of thousands of patients have benefited from this procedure. For the first time

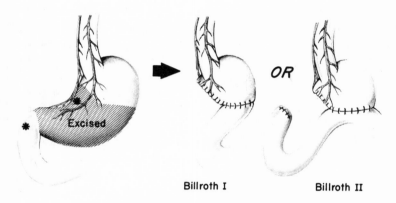

Billroth I   Billroth II

SUB-TOTAL GASTRECTOMY

Sixty-six to seventy-five percent of stomach removed and ends reattached in one of two ways. (Billroth I or II) Used for either duodenal or gastric ulcers.

an operation was available which brought cure in over 90 percent of the people operated on. Even more gratifying, when the operation was performed by competent surgeons, the mortality rate was reduced to less than 7 percent.

While sub-total gastrectomy was, and remains to this day, an excellent operation for ulcer, many now consider it to be insufficiently effective. Also, it is too dangerous when compared with newer and clearly better techniques, and a 7 percent mortality rate is now considered *much* too high. Therefore, despite the enormous contributions made by this operation, interest in it has sharply waned. Most surgeons trained during the last twenty years have largely abandoned it.

Sub-total gastrectomy is a paradox. The greater the amount of stomach removed, the more effective the cure. However, the price is a relatively high mortality rate and a high frequency of unpleasant side effects. The search continued for a safer, better tolerated and more effective operation.

In 1906, Edkins, an English physiologist, demonstrated that the antrum, the lower portion of the stomach, has a special function. It does not make acid; quite the contrary, it produces only mucus and the very important hormone he called gastrin. While physiologists were slow to recognize the validity of these observations, surgeons quickly learned to make use of them. Although Edkins's notion was initially thought incorrect and much abuse was heaped on his idea, it was subsequently proved to be valid. Then it became clear that only the upper part of the stomach (about 85 percent of it) was concerned with the making of acid. The lower part of the stomach was shown to be an endocrine organ like the thyroid or the adrenal glands, and its lining was primarily concerned with producing a stimulant to acid secretion.

Another observation contributed a key for the development of an operation that was to prove far more effective than the older procedures. During the early part of the nineteenth century it was noticed that dogs killed by an intravenous injection of arsenic, on postmortem examination, had an unusually large volume of mucus and water in their stomachs. It was also noted that if the vagus nerves were previously cut, the increased secretion of gastric juice seen after arsenic injection was prevented. Furthermore, in 1884 and again in 1910, Pavlov found failure of the digestive process in dogs in which the vagus nerves were cut.

An idea of tremendous importance was thus clearly established: the vagus nerves are critical in the normal carrying out of the stomach's muscular and secretory processes. Interruption of these nerves has a profound effect both on the ability of the stomach to empty itself and on its ability to make corrosive acid-pepsin juices.

This recognition of the importance of the vagus nerves, together with Edkins's description of the lower portion of the stomach as an endocrine organ helped pinpoint the two most important stimuli to stomach-acid secretion: the vagus nerves and the hormone gastrin. The foundation was laid for all modern surgery for peptic ulcer.

II. Vagotomy: On January 18, 1943, at the University of Chicago Clinic, Dragstedt * performed an operation in which the vagus nerves to the stomach were cut and no part of the stomach was removed. This procedure, widely referred to as a vagotomy, has become in one form or another the most important feature of present-day surgery for ulcers. Although others before Dragstedt had made smiliar attempts to cut the vagus nerves, poor appreciation of the somewhat difficult anatomy resulting in incomplete division of them, rendered these operations insufficiently effective.

But even Dragstedt's operation was not perfect. Cutting the vagus nerves to the stomach, while it does markedly reduce the production of acid juices, unfortunately has some unpleasant side effects. The vagus nerves are important not only in acid secretion, but also to the muscular activity of the stomach upon which normal emptying is dependent. It soon became apparent that in order to retain the beneficial effects of vagotomy (primarily decreased acid secretion) one must either widen the outlet of the stomach by cutting the muscular pyloric ring at its lower end, or make a new connection between the stomach and the lower intestine (see

* As a historical aside, Dragstedt was the surgeon later made famous by being the first to successfully separate Siamese twins.

Figure 5). These modifications helped compensate for the diminished strength of muscular propulsion of gastric contents.

These operations, now widely known as vagotomy and drainage procedures, are among the most popular used throughout the world today. This kind of surgery represents a significant advance over the partial removal of two-thirds of the stomach (sub-total gastrectomy) in that it is far safer and appears to have fewer side effects. Again, unfortunately, one

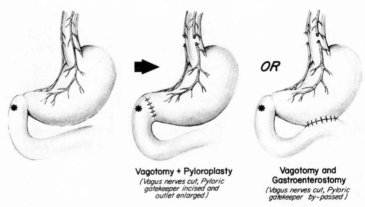

Vagotomy + Pyloroplasty
(Vagus nerves cut, Pyloric gatekeeper incised and outlet enlarged)

Vagotomy and Gastroenterostomy
(Vagus nerves cut, Pyloric gatekeeper by-passed)

VAGOTOMY AND DRAINAGE OPERATIONS FOR DUODENAL ULCER

pays a price for these advantages. Vagotomy and drainage, though safer, is somewhat less curative than the larger operation of sub-total gastrectomy.

The single most important consideration in surgery for peptic ulcer remains your safety. Cure rate, although it should be high, naturally takes second priority. Observations made on many thousands of patients treated by vagotomy and drainage have led to the conclusion that the operation is an extremely safe one. About 199 out of every 200 patients

SURGERY FOR PEPTIC ULCERS

tolerate it; side effects are minimal and well-handled; and approximately 92 to 93 percent of people so treated are cured and require no further therapy.

Ninety-nine to 99.5 percent safety is an outstanding improvement over the 93 percent safety factor observed after sub-total gastrectomy. But the 7 to 8 percent failure to cure became a new challenge, and the search for the perfect operation continued.

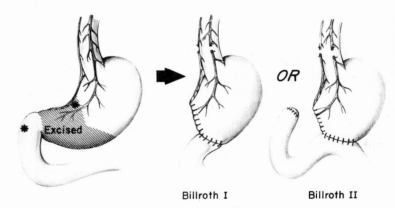

Billroth I   Billroth II

VAGOTOMY AND ANTRECTOMY
(Hemigastrectomy)

Forty to fifty percent of stomach removed and the vagus nerves cut. Ends reattached in one of two ways (Billroth I or II). Used for duodenal ulcers and sometimes for gastric ulcers.

III. Vagotomy and Antrectomy (or Hemigastrectomy): Since the two most important stimuli to acid secretion are the vagus nerves and the hormone gastrin, which is produced mostly in the antrum, it was suggested that an ideal operation would include removal of the antrum only, less tissue than is normally taken with sub-total gastrectomy, and cutting of the vagus nerves (see Figure 6). In 1947 Smithwick in Boston and Edwards in Nashville independently began performing this operation. The procedure, which has come to be known as vagotomy and antrectomy or vagotomy and hemigastrectomy, has been proved to be the most curative yet devised. Only about one patient in two hundred will fail to have his or her ulcer cured after this procedure. This is a truly remarkable record, and its consistency has been demonstrated and confirmed repeatedly in clinics throughout the world.

Although the cure rate is virtually perfect, the safety of the operation continues to be lessened by the surgical removal of part of the stomach, however limited. This operation is therefore slightly riskier than the vagotomy and drainage, though less risky than sub-total gastrectomy. The operation works the best but falls between the more extensive and less extensive procedures in terms of risk to life.

The search for the ideal operation—zero mortality, zero side effects and 100 percent cure rate—continues. A fourth operation, now being tested in clinics throughout the United States, Western Europe, Scandinavia and Great Britain holds promise for matching both the cure rate of hemigastrectomy and the safety of vagotomy and drainage. I have reserved detailed description of this operation for Chapter 16 because its use remains, for the present at least, in the realm of clinical experimental trial. For the most part the operations now being used for the treatment of duodenal and gastric ulcer are vagotomy and drainage or vagotomy and hemigastrectomy.

SELECTING THE PROPER OPERATION FOR AN INDIVIDUAL PATIENT

It is neither necessary nor desirable for all people undergoing surgery for peptic ulcer to have the same operation. I believe that a surgeon should not be committed to only one kind of operation for all people with ulcers. We now have enough data to tell us roughly which patients are at greatest risk from what operations; which operations can achieve the best cure rate, but at the expense of an increased ulcer recurrence. From the patient's point of view, we can also predict with some assurance who will tolerate which operation best in terms of side effects; who is likely to have a recurrence of an ulcer, despite surgery; who can "stand" undergoing the more major operation with the lowest risk and can reap the benefits of the highest cure rate without sacrifice of safety. Choosing the right operation for the right patient is as much an art as a science. In many respects this is what quality surgery is all about.

For some patients, particularly the very elderly or infirm, surgeons can accept a cure rate of only 90 to 93 percent in exchange for safety. For the younger and stronger patient with no complicating problems, we can afford to be more aggressive. We know that the more definitive operations are tolerated with safety by this group and we can attack the ulcer in a more certain fashion. By playing safety, curability, and freedom from side effects against age, other physical impairments and the virulence of a particular ulcer, we can attempt to do the best for the most.

Your safety is the most important consideration. It should never be compromised for curability. Although the recurrence rate after modern surgery is low, especially with the more aggressive operations, ulcers sometimes do return. Under these rare circumstances resumption of medical therapy or, more likely, a second operation may be required.

EPILOGUE ON SURGERY

A former teacher of mine, H. M. Spiro at Yale, has recently published a widely read and very authoritative textbook called *Diseases of the Gastrointestinal Tract*. In the chapter devoted to the management of peptic ulcer, he states: "Once an ulcer, always an ulcer." He goes on to say that "there is no way to cure an ulcer." What he really means, of course, is that there is no way to cure an ulcer with medication alone. Surgery cures.

Modern surgery is between 93 percent and 99.5 percent effective. The safety factor is in the 97.5 percent to 99.5 percent range. There are precious few things in this world of ours that work 93 to 99.5 percent of the time. Surgery for peptic ulcer is one of them.

It is a tribute to medical practice that surgeons do not consider these figures good enough. This is just as it should be. What we really want is a perfect operation—100 percent cure rate, no risks to life, and no discernible side effects. I am hopeful that we will have it one day. Certainly the hundred years since Rydygier's first attempt have brought us closer to our goal.

15

Life After Surgery

I would like to see the day when somebody would be appointed surgeon somewhere who had no hands, for the operative part is the least part of the work.

—Harvey Cushing (1869–1939)

The operation itself is but one incident, no doubt the most dramatic, yet still only one in the long series of events which must stretch between illness and recovery.

—Sir Berkley Moynihan (1865–1936)

By carefully selecting patients for operation and by tailoring the operation to the specific needs of the individual, surgeons maximize safety and minimize risk. Furthermore, surgery is safest and most effective when performed on a *planned* basis for almost all patients. If we don't think it will be, and our hand isn't forced by a complication such as bleeding or perforation, we won't recommend surgery. There are a few possible side effects of surgery you should be aware of and should know how to handle if they crop up.

THE TOO-SMALL STOMACH SYNDROME

Although the stomach is not essential to life, one of its primary functions is storage. An indefinable sensation referred to as the joy of having a stomach is lost when a large portion of the organ is removed. The privilege and pleasure of occasionally eating a large meal or overindulging without discomfort is certainly worth preserving.

The vagotomy and limited partial gastrectomy (vagotomy and hemigastrectomy) preserve this pleasure to a much greater extent than does a sub-total gastrectomy. Vagotomy and drainage, for practical purposes, preserves it completely. Getting full too quickly is not an important problem with the two modern operations. If you have had sub-total gastrectomy, and find yourself getting full too quickly, try eating smaller meals more frequently, up to six meals a day.

DUMPING

When the lower portion of the stomach is removed, or the pyloric sphincter (gate-keeper) is cut and enlarged, or a new opening is made between the stomach and the lower intestine, the ingenious mechanism that regulates gastric emptying is partially or completely lost. For most people this is not a serious problem, and within a year after operation they learn to adapt by cutting down on certain foods that contribute to a too-rapid emptying of the stomach.

The complex of symptoms that are a consequence of too-rapid emptying of the stomach are aptly called the "dumping syndrome." Foods and liquids that under normal circumstances are delivered in a regulated manner to the small intestine are now literally dumped directly into the upper bowel.

How to Handle Early Dumping: There are two variations of the dumping syndrome. The early postprandial (after meals) dumping syndrome occurs quite soon after eating foods rich in carbohydrates. Milkshakes, macaroni, thick gravy and thick soups, rich desserts and similar foods may cause dumping. The symptoms of dumping are not frightening nor life-threatening; they are simply unpleasant—sweating, rapid heartbeat, light-headedness, mild nausea and sometimes loose bowel movements.

In some extreme cases a dry diet works nicely. Don't take liquids with your meal; instead, wait until about a half-hour after eating. This is a very effective way to control dumping, and most people who suffer from dumping learn quickly how to successfully avoid it.

The incidence of dumping varies depending upon how much of your stomach is removed. If none of it is removed and only the outlet is interfered with, about one patient in seven will initially dump, and at the end of the first year after surgery only one patient in a hundred hasn't learned how to control it. When a small gastric resection has been carried out, up to one in five patients may dump. Once again, however, the symptoms are controllable by a common-sense approach to eating. Only under unusual circumstances does dumping incapacitate anyone for any length of time, and only rarely is further surgery required to correct this.

How to Handle Late Dumping: The late postprandial dumping syndrome results from low blood sugar (hypoglycemia), an overreaction by the pancreas to sugars introduced too rapidly into the small intestine, as in Naldo's case.

ST. LOUIS, MISSOURI. APRIL 25, 1977

Naldo is a thirty-eight-year-old Caucasian male postmaster in a rural branch post office. He underwent surgery for a duodenal ulcer fourteen months ago. His postoperative course was uncomplicated, his symptoms completely disappeared, and he's been enjoying life. He eats anything he wishes, including rich desserts.

About two months ago he noticed that an hour or two after eating a particularly rich meal he would feel lightheaded and would break into a cold sweat. His heart would beat rapidly. He's learned on his own that drinking a Coke quickly relieves the symptoms.

He's also gaining more weight than he'd like. He was advised to moderate his carbohydrate-rich diet and to carry a few pieces of hard candy in his pocket. Once he understood the cause of his symptoms, he could easily avoid them and rarely has to use the candy for relief. A less rich diet and a decreased need for sugar to relieve symptoms have allowed him to control his weight more easily.

In response to a sudden load of sugar placed in the small intestine, which is absorbed rapidly and makes its way quickly into the bloodstream, too much insulin pours from the pancreas, and the blood sugar drops sharply. The late postprandial dumping syndrome is a rare consequence of surgery, and I mention it primarily for completeness. People who suffer from it soon learn to carry a few pieces of chocolate or hard candy with them, so that if the symptoms occur, they can be rapidly and effectively gotten rid of.

CHANGES IN BOWEL HABITS

Most people who undergo duodenal ulcer surgery that involves cutting the vagus nerves experience changes in their bowel habits. In general, the tendency is toward a softer or looser bowel movement. The constipated patient may actually be happy with this side effect. The patient who prior to surgery usually had one or two bowel movements a day may not experience an increase in the number of stools, but they may be somewhat softer.

About 5 percent of vagotomy patients have two or more bowel movements a day after surgery, while about 1 percent may actually suffer from diarrhea that may require treatment. Some people who've had their vagus nerves cut experience what is called "episodic diarrhea," or more than two loose bowel movements per day once or twice a week. Again, this is not a serious problem, and most patients handle it very well.

We don't really understand why cutting the vagus nerves changes bowel habits. These nerves undoubtedly play an important role in the muscular activity of the intestine. But the fact that 95 percent of vagotomy patients don't suffer unpleasant consequences is confusing. Some observers feel that the decrease in the amount of acid produced in the stomach after an operation causes an imbalance in the bacteria that normally grow in the gastrointestinal tract. Others think that bile salt metabolism is altered and this causes looser stools, or that they result from changes in the nerve reflexes in the intestine. There are many theories, but none have been proven.

I am convinced that most of the time the urgent need to move the bowels is simply another form of dumping. Remarkable relief from this unpleasant side effect of surgery can be obtained by following the dry diet mentioned earlier. Avoid *all* liquids at mealtime. When liquids are mixed with food solids, the meal is simply dumped more easily and quickly into the intestines. Liquids also dissolve components of the food, particularly the sugars, and thus make it easier for them to be absorbed more rapidly by the intestine. This is a strong contributing factor to dumping and therefore to diarrhea.

After the dry meal is over, you can then have your coffee, tea or milk—but wait about a half-hour. Of course you can modify this regimen to meet your individual needs. I have found that this solves the problem most of the time.

MAINTENANCE OF NUTRITION

During the first year after a sub-total gastrectomy has been done, a significant percentage of patients lose six or more pounds and are not able to regain them. After the newer operations, however, most people maintain their weight or actually gain some, particularly if they were undernourished before the operation. The standard ulcer diet can be abandoned in the postoperative period, and patients can eat more normally.

I generally don't restrict the postoperative patient's diet once he or she has recovered and is out of the hospital. Some things you were able to eat or drink before your operation may now cause you some problems; many things which you couldn't eat before you can once again enjoy. I encourage patients to experiment with different foods and drinks and to determine for themselves what can be tolerated and what is best left alone. Even alcohol is usually no problem.

RECURRENCE OF ULCERS

The most vexing and disappointing postoperative problem is the development of a new ulcer or the failure of the old ulcer to heal. Fortunately, with such operations as vagotomy and hemigastrectomy, recurrence of ulcers is seen in only about one in two hundred people. The frequency of recurrence is higher with the less extensive vagotomy and drainage operation, but this is acceptable given the relative safety of the procedure, especially for the very old or infirm.

A common grading system for evaluating patients following surgery for peptic ulcers is the so-called Visick Classification. A modification of it consists of four categories:

Visick I: Perfect result. Ulcer cured. No side effects.

Visick II: Good result. Ulcer cured. Minimal side effects.

Visick III: Fair result. Ulcer cured. Moderate to severe side effects.

Visick IV: Poor result. Ulcer recurred or persists. Side effects severe and debilitating.

It is a measure of the quality of modern surgery that approximately 97 percent of patients (and 95 percent of physicians) report that the results of their operation for ulcers fall into either the Visick I or the Visick II categories. Surgery for peptic ulcer is extremely safe, very effective and well-tolerated. It can represent a true return to the joys of living and eating well.

16

New Approaches to Treatment

Be not the first by whom the new are tried,
Nor yet the last to lay the old aside.
—Alexander Pope (1688–1744),
An Essay on Criticism

Where our understanding of peptic ulcer and its medical and surgical control is concerned, there is every reason to believe that the best is yet to come. The primary role of medicine in society is not the successful treatment of disease, but the *prevention* of illness. However, until we do learn more about the causes of ulcer—and even more importantly, how to prevent them—we'll have to focus our attention on what the future holds for newer and better treatment.

HOPE FOR THE FUTURE IN THE MEDICAL MANAGEMENT OF ULCERS

We have recognized for a long time that synthetic histamine is a very powerful agent for stimulating the secretion of stomach acid. Naturally produced histamine may play a very important role as the final common pathway by which all other stimuli cause the stomach to produce acid. Whether the stomach is excited by emotional activity, with the vagus nerves as the pathway, or by hormonal activity as a result of the release of gastrin from the lower portion of the stomach, or by means of such agents as caffeine or alcohol, the last step in the stimulation of the stomach cells that secrete acid may depend on histamine.

Injection of histamine into experimental animals is a time-honored way to stimulate the stomach to maximally produce acid. Histamine has also been widely used in humans for the same purpose, in order to obtain a measure of the stomach's ability to produce acid. Usually, in the histamine test, an antihistamine is given about a half-hour before to help reduce such unpleasant side effects as a throbbing headache, facial flushing, sweating and a rapid heartbeat.

While the standard antihistamines effectively control the side effects of the drug, they do not have any apparent effect on its ability to stimulate the production of acid. These antihistamines block one effect of histamine but not the other. It has been theorized, based on these observations, that there are two receptors to histamine in the body, the H_1 receptor and the H_2 receptor. The H_1 receptor can be blocked by a standard antihistaminic compound. The remaining receptors, which control stomach-acid secretion and are not sensitive to antihistamines, are called H_2 receptors.

About fifteen years ago researchers at the Smith, Kline and French laboratories began to search for an effective H_2 receptor blocking agent. After almost eight years of intensive investigation a modification of the histamine molecule was constructed. Two compounds capable of blocking the H_2 receptors were developed.

These two drugs have considerable advantages over the old-style acid suppressors (anticholinergic drugs—see Chapter 12) because they don't cause certain unpleasant side effects—dryness of the mouth, blurring of vision, or difficulty in emptying the bladder. However, in the first tests on 150 humans, important toxic side effects *were* noticed, and these first drugs have been abandoned. Disappointment naturally was widespread. But the fact that the H_2 receptor had been identified and a synthetic agent had been produced to block it seemed reward enough for the effort and expense invested in the project.

In 1975 R. W. Brimbelcomb and his coworkers in New Zealand successfully synthesized a new drug that also resembled histamine, but that didn't seem to have any toxic side effects. This agent, called Cimetidine, is the newest and most exciting of the H_2 receptor antagonists. It can be taken orally and has been found to be as effective as its predecessors. It's in a class with the most powerful suppressors of acid and pepsin yet developed. It's effective against acid production stimulated by meals; it doesn't affect the emptying process of the stomach; and no side effects were observed in people with duodenal ulcers.

There is mounting evidence not only that the drug is useful in the relief of pain but also that it encourages healing of ulcers. And perhaps, with prolonged use, ulcer recurrences may be prevented. It may well be "a pharmacological dream come true."

Naturally, much more extensive clinical testing, as well as experimental study, must be carried out before the safety and effectiveness of this drug can be established. It will take years, and thousands of people with ulcers will have to be observed before reliable data can be accumulated. However, even if Cimetidine isn't the ultimate H_2 receptor blocker, the trail has clearly been blazed.

HOPE FOR THE FUTURE IN ULCER SURGERY

We know that the vagus nerves carry impulses that are extremely important in the stimulation and control of the stomach's ability to secrete acid. One unfortunate side effect of cutting the vagus nerves has been that the stomach's ability to empty itself can be impaired, causing postoperative problems. A number of operations have been designed to compensate the stomach for this decreased muscle tone and still permit the beneficial acid-suppressing features of vagotomy. These operations have proven to be extremely effective and for the most part do their job well. On the other hand, some side effects of these operations prevent them from being perfect.

Although the entire stomach plays a role in mixing and propelling food through the pyloric outlet, the most important part of this mechanism is found in the antrum. Preservation of the pyloric ring at the lower end of the stomach is important in regulating the rate at which the stomach empties. A more perfect operation would preserve the mixing and emptying functions of the stomach but reduce acid secretion.

Such an operation has been devised and is now undergoing widespread clinical trial throughout the United States, Scandinavia, Western Europe and Great Britain. The procedure, called a highly selective vagotomy, preserves the fibers of the vagus nerves that control the muscular activity at the lower end of the stomach, but cuts those fibers that primarily affect acid secretion. It is still far too early to fully assess the effectiveness of this operation, but this procedure is clearly the safest of all the operations yet devised, and with the exception of only a very few cases among the more than 5,500 operations performed to date, it involves no risk.

The operation is technically difficult and tedious compared to the other operations in common use. Until surgeons throughout the world learn to carry out the operation properly it probably won't have any significant advantages over the other two procedures—vagotomy and drainage and vagotomy and hemigastrectomy—now in widespread use.

Nevertheless, since surgery for duodenal ulcers is the only

known permanent cure, advances in surgical technique are very important. The hope, therefore, is that with refinement, highly selective vagotomy will eventually prove to be the most effective, the safest and the freest from side effects of all surgical techniques for dealing with ulcer. If not, the search for the perfect surgical cure will continue.

CENTER FOR ULCER RESEARCH AND EDUCATION (CURE)

As befits one of our most important public health problems, a Center for Ulcer Research and Education was established in April 1974 under the direction of Morton I. Grossman, M.D., Ph.D., one of the most distinguished gastric physiologists in the world. CURE's goals are to gain new knowledge about peptic ulcer and to disseminate this knowledge to doctors, patients and the general public. It is expected that CURE will generate information that will lead to improved prevention, diagnosis, and medical and surgical treatment of peptic ulcers.

CURE provides a crucible with the diverse talents of highly-qualified scientists from many different disciplines interacting. Some of these disciplines are not conventionally regarded as being related to research on peptic ulcer. Most of CURE's studies involve the collaborative efforts of two or more key investigators.

Over one hundred publications have resulted thus far from this extraordinarily diverse and productive group of scientists—epidemiologists, physiologists, anatomists, surgeons, biochemists, geneticists, biophysicists, pediatricians, gastroenterologists, neurophysiologists, immunologists and others. This massive joint effort, partially supported by the Veterans' Administration and by grants from the National Institute of Arthritis, Metabolism and Digestive Diseases, together with the efforts of thousands of others all over the world, must surely one day bring our understanding of ulcers to the point where we can not only cure them, but prevent them as well.

Afterword

Heredity sets limits, environment decides the exact position within these limits.

—E. C. MacDowell (1887–   )

You are now aware—in fact, you probably always knew—that peptic ulcer is an extremely complicated disorder. The geneticist sees ulcers as an inherited problem. The psychiatrist views them in terms of personality. The environmentalist puts heaviest emphasis on the individual response to the "world without," while the physiologist stresses the "world within." I tend to think of the factors involved in causing ulcers as pieces in a jigsaw puzzle. Some fit together neatly and form a larger fragment of our understanding; some obviously are part of the puzzle, but where they should be placed is not yet clear; some pieces appear to be missing altogether.

Ulcers develop not from one but from a constellation of forces. They arise in a setting, a fertile soil into which a "bad seed" falls and germinates to produce one of mankind's most unpleasant ailments. We know something about this very receptive soil.

If you're a male; if you have blood group type O; if you can't secrete the blood group antigens in your saliva; if you have a family history of ulcers; if you make higher than normal amounts of acid and pepsin; if you're a female going through the menopause; and so on, you are a particularly vulnerable target for ulcers. If you then experience some kind of stress—for example, conflicts within yourself—ulcers can result.

Some stresses and conflicts are under our control; others are not. Your job may be one of them. Another may be divorce, bankruptcy, loss of a mate or child, an illness or an operation, a thwarted ambition, a loss of self-esteem, or even a war. But what seems most important is how you perceive or handle your own private hell. If you make a fist in your pocket, if you grin and bear it, if you perpetually keep a "stiff upper lip"—if, in other words, you turn your anguish *in*—you may be doing yourself a disservice.

When we are truly happy we smile and we laugh. This is a perfectly acceptable and rational response to pleasure. Why, then, when we are unhappy, do we so often suppress our true feelings? Appropriate anger—controlled, but anger nevertheless—is healthy and sometimes cleansing. Angering-out may not prevent ulcers, but it's a beginning.

In his textbook entitled *Clinical Gastroenterology*, H. M. Spiro relates this story of a physician who demonstrates the possible protective aspect of an "anger-out" personality:

NEW HAVEN, CONNECTICUT. FEBRUARY 15, 1969

Francis is a forty-year-old practicing physician. For many years he had the reputation of being a curmudgeon and was known to chase some patients from his office, give salty advice to others, and generally was prone to raise cain. Six months ago he had decided that it was time for a change. He would become sweetness and light, and, life being short, he would be kind to everyone, regardless of how he really felt.

On precisely the day that he made that decision, he first suffered severe ulcer pain. Within a few weeks it progressed in severity and began to penetrate through to his back. Ultimately, he was admitted to the hospital with "intractable" pain, unrelieved by medications. A duodenal ulcer that had penetrated through the back wall and was eroding into the pancreas was diagnosed. He faced the decision as to whether or not surgery was required.

When confronted with the reality and possibility of an operation he recognized exactly what had happened and what his cure should be. Soon after discharge from the hospital, he resumed his more traditional caustic and dour behavior, and the ulcer for which operation seemed so inevitable stopped causing him pain. It has not recurred.

Whether or not this story is true I have no way of knowing. But if it isn't, it ought to be.

It would be dangerous, or misleading at best, to oversimplify the causes of ulcer, or how to prevent them. Attention to diet, moderation in coffee, tea, alcohol and tobacco consumption, avoidance of aspirin, and change of occupation can all be of possible help in preventing ulcers or managing them if they are already present. A common-sense approach to life is a realistic goal.

It would be easy for me to indict the frenzied environment we live in as an important cause of ulcers. Unfortunately, the data aren't solid. The frequency of ulcers is rising again, but no clear-cut relationship to today's fast pace of life has been proven. What I do know is that regardless of the outside world, your response to it is what counts. The important difference between those who have ulcers and those who don't rests within. Don't drop out—fight back.

Sources and Supplementary Reading

Aird, I. "Discussion on the ABO Blood Groups and Disease."
Proceedings of the Royal Society of Medicine 48:139, 1955.
————, H.H. Bentall, and J.A.F. Roberts. "Relationships Between Cancer of the Stomach and ABO Blood Groups."
British Medical Journal 1:799, 1953.
Alexander, F. "The Influence of Psychologic Factors Upon Gastrointestinal Disturbances." *Psychiatric Quarterly* 3:501, 1934.
————. *Psychosomatic Medicine.* New York: Norton, 1950.
Almy, T.P., Panel Moderator. "Prevalence and Significance of Digestive Disease." *Gastroenterology* 68:1351, 1975.
Alp, M.H., J.H. Court, and K.A. Grant. "Personality Pattern and Emotional Stress in the Genesis of Gastric Ulcer." *Gut* 11:773, 1970.
Alsted, G. *The Changing Incidence of Peptic Ulcer.* London: Oxford University Press, 1939.
————. "The Social and Public Health Aspect of Peptic Ulcer." *Gastroenterology* 26:268, 1954.

SOURCES AND SUPPLEMENTARY READING

Alvey, C., and A. Cahn. "Orange Juice and Digestive Dysfunction." *Medical Journal of Australia* 2:11, 1956.

Amdrup, E., and H.E. Jensen. "Selective Vagotomy of the Parietal Cell Mass Preserving Innervation of the Undrained Antrum." *Gastroenterology* 59:522, 1970.

American Dietetic Association Position Paper on Bland Diet in the Treatment of Chronic Duodenal Ulcer Disease. Approved by the Executive Board May 21, 1971.

Apter, A., and L.A. Hurst. "Personality and Duodenal Ulcer." *South African Medical Journal* 47:2131, 1973.

Backus, F.I., and D.L. Dudley. "Observations of Psychosocial Factors and Their Relationship to Organic Disease." *International Journal of Psychiatry in Medicine* 5:499, 1974.

Banks, C.N., and J.H. Baron "Drugs Containing Aspirin." *Lancet* 1:1165, 1964.

Baron, J.H. "Peptic Ulcer, Gastric Secretion and Body Build." *Gut* 5:83, 1964.

Barreras, R.F. "Acid Secretion After Calcium Carbonate in Patients with Duodenal Ulcer." *New England Journal of Medicine* 282:1402, 1970.

Beaumont, W. *Experiments and Observations on the Gastric Juice and the Physiology of Digestion.* New York: Dover, 1959 (originally published in 1833).

Becker, K.L. "Genetic Aspects of Gastrointestinal Disease." *Medical Clinics of North America* 52:1273, 1968.

Belker, J.P. "Gastroscopy and Duodenoscopy." In M.H. Sleisenger and J.S. Fordtran, eds., *Gastrointestinal Disease.* Philadelphia: W.B. Saunders, 1973.

Bennett, J.R. "Progress Report: Smoking and the Gastrointestinal Tract." *Gut* 13:658, 1972.

Billington, B.P. "Observations from New South Wales on the Changing Incidence of Gastric Ulcer in Australia." *Gut* 6:121, 1965.

Black, J.W., W.A.M. Duncan, C.J. Durant et al. "Definition and Antagonism of Histamine H_2 Receptors." *Nature* (London) 236:385, 1972.

Blumenthal, I.S. *The Social Cost of Peptic Ulcer.* Santa Monica, Calif.: Rand Corporation, 1967.

Bock, O.A.A. "Alcohol, Aspirin, Depression, Smoking, Stress and

SOURCES AND SUPPLEMENTARY READING

the Patient with a Gastric Ulcer." *South African Medical Journal* 50:293, 1976.

Boley, S.J., H. Krieger, S. Schwartz et al. "The Effect of Operations for Peptic Ulcer on Growth and Nutrition of Puppies." *Surgery* 57:441, 1965.

Brady, J.V. "Ulcers in 'Executive Monkeys.'" *Scientific American* 199:95, 1958.

Brimblecombe, R.W., W.A.M. Duncan, G.J. Durant et al. "Cimetidine—A Non-Thiourea H_2-Receptor Antagonist." *Journal of Internal Medicine Research* 3:86, 1975.

Brown, D.A., A.G.P. Melrose, and J. Wallace. "The Blood Groups in Peptic Ulceration." *British Medical Journal* 2:135, 1956.

Buchman, E., D. Kaung, K. Dolan, and R. Knapp. "Unrestricted Diet in the Treatment of Duodenal Ulcer." *Gastroenterology* 56:1010, 1969.

————, ————, and R. Knapp. "Dietary Treatment in Duodenal Ulcer." *American Journal of Clinical Nutrition* 22:1536, 1969.

Buckwalter, J.A., et al. "Peptic Ulceration and ABO Blood Groups." *Journal of the American Medical Association* 162:1215, 1956.

Camerer, J.W. *Zeitschrift fuer Menschliche Vererbungs und Konstitutionslehre* 19:416, 1935.

Cameron, A.D. "Gastrointestinal Blood Loss Measured by Radioactive Chromium." *Gut* 1:177, 1960.

Cannon, W. *Bodily Changes in Pain, Hunger, Fear and Rage.* New York: Appleton-Century-Crofts, 1929.

Card, W.I., and I.N. Marks. "The Relationship Between the Acid Output of the Stomach Following 'Maximal' Histamine Stimulation and the Parietal Cell Mass." *Clinical Science and Molecular Medicine* 19:147, 1960.

Chapman, B.L., and J.M. Duggan. "Environmental Factors and the Australian Gastric Ulcer Change." *Medical Journal of Australia* 1:1179, 1969.

Chen, E., and S. Cobb. "Family Structure in Relation to Health and Disease. A Review of the Literature." *Journal of Chronic Diseases* 12:544, 1960.

Chuttani, P.N., and A.K. Sehgal. "Incidence of Peptic Ulcer in the Punjab." *Journal of the Association of Physicians of India* 6:347, 1958.

Clark, D.H. "Peptic Ulcer in Women." *British Medical Journal* 1:1254, 1953.

Clarke, C.A., et al. "The Relationship of ABO Blood Groups to Duodenal and Gastric Ulceration." *British Medical Journal* 1:643, 1955.

————, C.A. Evans, D.A.P. Evans, et al. "Secretion of Blood Group Antigens and Peptic Ulcer." *British Medical Journal* 1:603, 1959.

Coddington, R.D. "Study on an Infant with a Gastric Fistula and Her Normal Twin." *Psychosomatic Medicine* 30:172, 1968.

Code, C.F. "Stimulating Effects of Various Foods on Gastric-Acid Secretion." *American Journal of Digestive Diseases* 6:50, 1953.

"Coffee Drinking and Peptic Ulcer Disease." *Nutritional Reviews* 34:167, 1976.

Cohen, S., and G.H. Booth, Jr. "Gastric Acid Secretion and Lower-Esophageal-Sphincter Pressure in Response to Coffee and Caffeine." *New England Journal of Medicine* 293:897, 1975.

Cohen, S.I., A.J. Silverman, and F. Magnusson. "New Psychophysiologic Correlates in Women with Peptic Ulcer." *American Journal of Psychiatry* 112:1025, 1956.

Comfort, M.W., H.K. Gray, M.B. Dockerty et al. "Small Gastric Cancer." *Archives of Internal Medicine* 94:513, 1954.

Cooper, P., and S.H. Tolins. "Relationship Between Smoking History and Complications Immediately Following Surgery for Duodenal Ulcer." *Mount Sinai Journal of Medicine* 39(3):287, 1972.

Crider, R.J., and S.M. Walker. "Physiologic Studies on the Stomach of a Woman with a Gastric Fistula." *A.M.A. Archives of Surgery* 57:1, 1948.

Csato, T. "Peptic Ulcer in Women." Correspondence. *British Medical Journal* 2:95, 1953.

Cushing, H. "Peptic Ulcers and the Interbrain." *Surgery, Gynecology and Obstetrics* 55:1, 1932.

D'Alonzo, C.A., D.M. Densen, A.J. Fleming, and M.J. Munn.

SOURCES AND SUPPLEMENTARY READING

"The Prevalence of Certain Diseases Among Executives in Comparison with Other Employees." *Industrial Medicine* 23:357, 1954.

Damon, A., and A.P. Palednak. "Constitution, Genetics and Body Form in Peptic Ulcer. A Review." *Journal of Chronic Diseases* 20:787, 1967.

Davenport, H.W. "Salicylate Damage to the Gastric Mucosal Barrier." *New England Journal of Medicine* 276:1307, 1967.

Debas, H.T., M.M. Cohen, I.B. Holubitzky, and R.C. Harrison. "Effect of Cigarette Smoking on Human Gastric Secretory Responses." *Gut* 12:93, 1971.

Demole, M.J., and G. Hecker. "Seasonal Periodicity of Duodenal Ulcer. A Statistical Study." *Gastroenterologia* 105:82, 1966.

Doll, R., F. Avery-Jones, and M. Buckatzsch. *Occupational Factors in the Etiology of Gastric and Duodenal Ulcers.* London: His Majesty's Stationery Office, 1951.

————, ————, and F. Pygott. "Effect of Smoking on the Production and Maintenance of Gastric and Duodenal Ulcer." *Lancet* 1:657, 1958.

————, and J. Buch. "Hereditary Factors in Peptic Ulcer." *Annals of Eugenics* 15:135, 1950.

————, and T.D. Kellock. "The Separate Inheritance of Gastric and Duodenal Ulcers." *Annals of Eugenics* 16:231, 1951.

Donaldson, R.M. "The Muddle of Diets for Gastrointestinal Disorders." *Journal of the American Medical Association* 225:1243, 1973.

Draper, G. *Human Constitution: Its Significance in Medicine and How It May Be Studied.* Beaumont Foundation Lecture Series No. 7. Baltimore: Williams & Wilkins, 1928.

Duggan, J.M. "Progress Report: Aspirin in Chronic Gastric Ulcer: An Australian Experience." *Gut* 17:378, 1976.

————, and B.L. Chapman. "The Incidence of Aspirin Ingestion in Patients with Peptic Ulcer." *Medical Journal of Australia,* 57(1B):797, April 18, 1970.

Dunn, J.P., and S. Cobb. "Frequency of Peptic Ulcer Among Executives, Craftsmen and Foremen." *Journal of Occupational Medicine* 4:343, 1962.

Eagle, P.C., and J. Gillman. "The Incidence of Peptic Ulcer in the South African Bantu." *South African Journal of Medical Science* 616:33, 1937.

Earlam, R. "A Computerized Questionnaire Analysis of Duodenal Ulcer Symptoms." *Gastroenterology* 71:314, 1976.

Eberhard, G. "Peptic Ulcer in Twins: A Study in Personality, Heredity, and Environment." *Acta Psychiatrica Scandinavica* 44, Supplement 205, 1968.

"Editorial: Children with Peptic Ulceration." *British Medical Journal,* 1:584, 1970.

Eichhorn, R., and J. Tractir. "The Effect of Hypnosis Upon Gastric Secretion." *Gastroenterology* 29:417, 1955.

————, and ————. "The Relationship Between Anxiety, Hyperatically Induced Emotions, and Gastric Secretion." *Gastroenterology* 29:422, 1955.

Einhorn, M. "Suspenders vs. Belts in Treatment of Gastric and Duodenal Ulcers." *American Journal of Medical Science* 175:395, 1928.

Eisenberg, M.M. "Physiologic Approach to the Surgical Management of Duodenal Ulcer." In *Current Problems in Surgery XIV*. Chicago: Year Book Medical Publishers, 1977.

————, J.E. Owens, and E.R. Woodward. "Effects of a Synthetic Androgen (TCPP) on Denervated Canine Gastric Pouches." *American Surgeon* 31:135, 1965.

————, and E.R. Woodward. "A Physiologic Approach to the Surgical Treatment of Peptic Ulcer." In J.H. Davis, ed., *Current Concepts in Surgery*. New York: McGraw-Hill, 1965.

Ellis, M. "A Study of Peptic Ulcer in Nigeria." *British Journal of Surgery* 36:60, 1948.

Engel, G.L. "The Concept of Psychosomatic Disease." *Journal of Psychosomatic Research* 11:1, 1967.

————. "Guilt, Pain and Success." *Psychosomatic Medicine* 24:37, 1962.

————. "Peptic Ulcer: Psychophysiological Gastrointestinal Disorders." In Syllabus of Postgraduate Course on Peptic Ulcer Disease, American Gastroenterological Association. Co-directors J.I. Isenberg and J.C. Thompson. San Francisco, May 19–20, 1974.

SOURCES AND SUPPLEMENTARY READING

————. " 'Psychogenic' Pain and the Pain-Prone Patient." *American Journal of Medicine* 26:899, 1959.

————, F. Reichsman, and H.L. Segal. "A Study of an Infant with a Gastric Fistula. I. Behavior and the Rate of Total Hydrochloric Acid Secretion." *Psychosomatic Medicine* 18: 374, 1956.

Falconer, D.S. "The Inheritance of Liability to Certain Diseases, Estimated from the Incidence Among Relatives." *Annals of Human Genetics* 29:51, 1965.

Fordtran, J.S. "Acid Rebound." *New England Journal of Medicine* 279:900, 1968.

————. "Acid Secretion in Peptic Ulcer." In M.H. Sleisenger and J.S. Fordtran, eds., *Gastrointestinal Disease*. Philadelphia: W.B. Saunders, 1973.

————. "The Psychosomatic Theory of Peptic Ulcer." In M.H. Sleisenger and J.S. Fordtran, eds., *Gastrointestinal Disease*. Philadelphia: W.B. Saunders, 1973.

————. "Reduction of Acidity by Diet, Antacids, and Anticholinergic Agents." In M.H. Sleisenger and J.S. Fordtran, eds., *Gastrointestinal Disease*. Philadelphia: W.B. Saunders, 1973.

————, S.G. Morawski, and C.T. Richardson. "In Vivo and In Vitro Evaluation of Liquid Antacids." *New England Journal of Medicine* 288:923, 1973.

Freud, S. "Analysis: Terminable and Interminable." In Vol. 5 of the *Collected Works*. London: Hogarth Press, 1950 (originally published in 1937).

Friedman, G.D., M.S. Siegelaub, and C.C. Seltzer. "Cigarettes, Alcohol, Coffee and Peptic Ulcer." *New England Journal of Medicine* 290:469, 1974.

Gardiner, G.C., W. Pinsky, and R.M. Meyerson. "The Seasonal Incidence of Peptic Ulcer Activity—Fact or Fancy?" *American Journal of Gastroenterology* 45:22, 1966.

Goldberg, E.M. *Family Influences and Psychosomatic Illness*. London: Tavistock, 1958.

Goldberg, H.I. "Roentgen Diagnosis of Ulcerative Diseases." In M.H. Sleisenger and J.S. Fordtran, eds., *Gastrointestinal Disease*. Philadelphia: W.B. Saunders, 1973.

Goldberg, H.M. "Duodenal Ulcers in Children." *British Medical Journal* 1:1500, 1957.

SOURCES AND SUPPLEMENTARY READING

Goldberg, S.J., C.L. Smith, and A.M. Connell. "Emotion-Related Gastritis." *American Journal of Gastroenterology* 65:41, 1976.

Grayson, R.R. "Air Controllers Syndrome: Peptic Ulcer in Air Traffic Controllers." *Illinois Medical Journal* 2:111, 1972.

Griffith, C.A., and H.N. Harkins. "Partial Gastric Vagotomy: An Experimental Study." *Gastroenterology* 32:96, 1957.

Groen, J. *De Psychopathogenese van het ulcus Ventriculi et Duodeni.* Amsterdam: Scheltema en Holkema.

Groen, J.J. "The Psychosomatic Specificity Hypothesis for the Etiology of Peptic Ulcer." *Psychotherapy and Psychosomatics* 19:295, 1971.

Grossman, M.I. CURE Brochure. Veterans Administration Wadsworth Hospital Center Building 115, Los Angeles, California.

————. "Duration of Action of Antacids." *American Journal of Digestive Diseases* 1:453, 1956.

————, Moderator. "A New Look at Peptic Ulcer: Panel Discussion." *Annals of Internal Medicine* 84:57, 1976.

————, and S.J. Konturek. "Inhibition of Acid Secretion in Dog by Metiamide, a Histamine Antagonist Acting on H_2 Receptors." *Gastroenterology* 66:517, 1974.

Habbick, B.F., A.G. Melrose, and Grant. "Duodenal Ulcer in Childhood. A Study of Predisposing Factors." *Archives of Disease in Childhood* 43:23, 1968.

Hadley, G.G. "A Study of Peptic Ulcer as Found in South India." Indian Council of Medicine Research Report, 1959.

Haggard, H.W., and L.A. Greenberg. "The Influence of Certain Fruit Juices on Gastric Function." *American Journal of Digestive Diseases* 8:163, 1941.

Hagnell, O., and G. Wretmark. "Peptic Ulcer and Alcoholism." *Journal of Psychosomatic Research* 2:35, 1957.

Halsted, J., and H. Weinberg. "Peptic Ulcer Among Soldiers in the Mediterranean Theater of Operations." *New England Journal of Medicine* 234:313, 1946.

Hamperl, H. "Ergebnisse der Allgemeine Pathologie und Pathologie." *Anatomie* 26:353, 1932.

Hansen, J.L. *Aendringer; ulcussydommens frem traeden.* Copenhagen: Ejnar Munksgaard, 1943.

Harkins, H.N., and L.M. Nyhus. *Surgery of the Stomach and Duodenum.* Boston: Little, Brown, 1962.

SOURCES AND SUPPLEMENTARY READING

Harvald, B., and M. Hauge. "Hereditary Factors Elucidated by Twin Studies." In J.V. Neel, M.W. Shaw and W.J. Schull, eds., *Genetics and the Epidemiology of Chronic Diseases.* U.S. Public Health Service Publication No. 1163. Washington, D.C.: U.S. Government Printing Office, 1965.

Herrington, J.L., Jr. "Current Operations for Duodenal Ulcer." In *Current Problems in Surgery.* Chicago: Year Book Medical Publishers, July 1972.

Hoelzel, F., and E. DeCosta. "Production of Peptic Ulcers in Rats and Mice by Diets Deficient in Protein." *American Journal of Digestive Diseases* 4:325, 1937.

Højer-Pedersen, W. "On the Significance of Psychic Factors in the Development of Peptic Ulcer." *Acta Psychiatrica Scandinavica* Supplement 119, 1958.

Holle, F., and S. Andersson, eds. *Vagotomy, Latest Advances.* New York: Springer-Verlag, 1974.

————, and W. Hart. "Neue Wege der Chirurgie des Gastroduodenal Ulkus." *Meizinische Klinik* 62:441, 1967.

Hussar, A.E. "Peptic Ulcer in Long-term Institutionalized Schizophrenic Patients." *Psychosomatic Medicine* 20:374, 1968.

Ingelfinger, F.J. "Anticholinergic Therapy of Gastrointestinal Disorders." *New England Journal of Medicine* 268:1454, 1963.

————. "Let the Ulcer Patient Enjoy His Food." In F.J. Ingelfinger et al., eds., *Controversy in Internal Medicine.* Philadelphia: W.B. Saunders, 1966.

Isenberg, J.I. "Gastric Secretory Testing." In M.H. Sleisenger and J.S. Fordtran, eds., *Gastrointestinal Disease.* Philadelphia: W.B. Saunders, 1973.

————. "H_2-Receptor Antagonists in the Treatment of Peptic Ulcer." *Annals of Internal Medicine* 84:212, 1976.

Ivy, A.C., M.I. Grossman, and W.H. Bachrach. *Peptic Ulcer.* New York: Blakiston/McGraw-Hill, 1950.

Jackson, R.H. "Genetic Factors in the Development of Duodenal Ulcer in Childhood." *Gut* 12:856, 1971.

Janowitz, H.D., M.H. Levy, and F. Hollander. "Diagnostic Significance of Urinary Pepsinogen Excretion in Diseases of the Upper Gastrointestinal Tract." *American Journal of Medical Science* 220:679, 1950.

SOURCES AND SUPPLEMENTARY READING

Jedrychowski, W., and T. Popiela. "Association Between the Occurrence of Peptic Ulcers and Tobacco Smoking." *Public Health* (London) 88:195, 1974.

Johnson, R.B., D.M. McCance, and W.M. Lukash. "Coffee—Trick or Treat?" *American Family Physician* 6:101, 1975.

Johnston, D., and A.R. Wilkinson. "Highly Selective Vagotomy Without a Drainage Procedure in the Treatment of Duodenal Ulcer." *British Journal of Surgery* 57:289, 1970.

Juniper, K. "The Relative Effective Dose of an Anticholinergic Drug, Glycopyrrolate, on Basal Gastric Secretion and Sweat and Salivary-gland Activity." *American Journal of Digestive Diseases* 12:439, 1967.

Kalk, H. *Das Magen und Zwölffingerdarm Geschwür im Kriege.* Leipzig: G. Thieme, 1945.

Kapp, F.T., M. Rosenbaum, and J. Romano. "Psychological Factors in Men with Peptic Ulcers." *American Journal of Psychiatry* 103:700, 1947.

Kehoe, M., and W. Ironside. "Studies on the Experimental Evocation of Depressive Responses Using Hypnosis. II. The Influence of Depressive Responses Upon the Secretion of Gastric Acid." *Psychosomatic Medicine* 25:403, 1963.

Kellock, T.D. "Childhood Factors in Duodenal Ulcer." *British Medical Journal* 2:1117, 1951.

Kezur, E., F.T. Kapp, and M. Rosenbaum. "Psychological Factors in Women with Peptic Ulcers." *American Journal of Psychiatry* 108:368, 1951.

Kimball, S. "Heredity and Peptic Ulcer." In D.J. Sandweiss, ed., *Peptic Ulcer.* Philadelphia: W.B. Saunders, 1951.

Kirsner, J.B. "Drug-Induced Peptic Ulcer." *Annals of Internal Medicine* 47:666, 1957.

————, and W.L. Palmer. "The Effect of Various Antacids on the Hydrogen-ion Concentration of the Gastric Contents." *American Journal of Digestive Diseases* 7:85, 1940.

Klinge, G.G., and L. Peña. "The Gastroduodenal Ulcer in High Altitudes (Peruvian Andes)." *Gastroenterology* 37:390, 1959.

Konstam, P.G. "Peptic Ulcer in Southern Nigeria." *Lancet* 2:1039, 1954.

Kral, V.A. "Psychiatric Observations Under Severe Chronic Stress." *American Journal of Psychiatry* 108:185, 1951.

SOURCES AND SUPPLEMENTARY READING

Kramer, P., and E.K. Caso. "Is the Rationale for Gastrointestinal Dietary Therapy Sound?" *Journal of the American Dietetic Association* 42:505, 1963.

Kretchmar, M. "Recrudescence of Gastroduodenal Ulcer in the Course of 1939–44 and the War-time Diet." *Gastroenterologia* 70:225, 1945.

Langman, M.J.S. "Epidemiological Evidence for the Association of Aspirin and Acute Gastrointestinal Bleeding." *Gut* 11: 627, 1970.

Lennard-Jones, J.E., and N. Barbouris. "Effect of Different Foods on the Acidity of Gastric Contents in Patients with Duodenal Ulcer. Part I. A Comparison Between Two 'Therapeutic' Diets and Freely Chosen Meals." *Gut* 6:113, 1965.

The Liquor Handbook. New York: Gavis-Jobson Associates, 1976.

Mahl, G.F. "Anxiety, HCI Secretion, and Peptic Ulcer Etiology." *Psychosomatic Medicine* 3:158, 1950.

Margolin, S.G. "The Behavior of the Stomach During Psychoanalysis." *Psychoanalytic Quarterly* 20:347, 1951.

Markoff, N. "Liegt eine Zunhame der Magendarmkrankheiten in der jetzigen Zeit vor?" *Gastroenterologia* 68:225, 1943.

Maxwell, J.C., Jr. "Low Tar Brands Heading for 20% of Total Cigarette Market." *Tobacco International,* November 26, 1976, p. 19.

McConnell, R.B. "Progress Report: Genetics and Gastroenterology." *Gut* 12:592, 1971.

Meade, T.W., T.H.D. Arie, M. Brewis et al. "Recent History of Ischemic Heart Disease and Duodenal Ulcer in Doctors." *British Medical Journal* 3:701, 1968.

Mendeloff, A.I. "What Has Been Happening to Duodenal Ulcer." *Gastroenterology* 67:1020, 1974.

————. "Epidemiology of Gastric Ulcer." Postgraduate Course on Peptic Ulcer Disease, Proceedings. American Gastroenterological Association, San Francisco, 1974.

Menguy, R. *Surgery of Peptic Ulcer.* Philadelphia: W.B. Saunders, 1976.

Metzger, Wm. H., L. McAdam, R. Bluestone, and P.H. Guth. "Acute Gastric Mucosal Injury During Continuous or Interrupted Aspirin Ingestion in Humans." *American Journal of Digestive Diseases* 21:963, 1976.

SOURCES AND SUPPLEMENTARY READING

Mirsky, I.A. "Physiologic, Psychologic and Social Determinants in the Etiology of Duodenal Ulcer." *American Journal of Digestive Diseases* 3:285, 1958.

Mittleman, B., and H.G. Wolff. "Emotions and Gastroduodenal Function: Experimental Studies on Patients with Gastritis, Duodenitis and Peptic Ulcer." *Psychosomatic Medicine* 4:5, 1942.

Monson, R.R. "Cigarette Smoking and Body Form in Peptic Ulcer." *Gastroenterology* 58:337, 1970.

———. "Familial Factors in Peptic Ulcer I. The Occurrence of Ulcer in Relatives." *Journal of Epidemiology* 91:453, 1970.

———, and B. MacMahon. "Peptic Ulcer in Massachusetts Physicians." *New England Journal of Medicine* 281:11, 1969.

Morgan, R.H., and M.W. Donner. "The Roentgenologic Diagnosis of Diseases of the Gastrointestinal Tract." In M. Paulson, ed., *Gastroenterologic Medicine*. Philadelphia: Lea & Febiger, 1969.

Necheles, H. "Peptic Ulcer in the Chinese." *American Journal of Digestive Diseases* 6:50, 1939.

Novis, B.H., I.N. Marks, S. Bank, and A.W. Sloan. "The Relation Between Gastric Acid Secretion and Body Habits, Blood Groups, Smoking, and the Subsequent Development of Dyspepsia and Duodenal Ulcer." *Gut* 14:107, 1973.

Nuss, D., and H.B. Lynn. "Peptic Ulceration in Childhood." *Surgical Clinics of North America* 51:945, 1971.

Ontaneda, M. "Biological-Psychological-Social Factors in Genesis of Peptic Ulcer." *American Journal of Proctology* 19:55, 1968.

Oshsner, A. "Treatment of Peptic Ulcer Disease." In R.L. Varco and J.P. Delaney, eds., *Controversy in Surgery*. Philadelphia: W.B. Saunders, 1976.

Paffenbarger, R.S., A.L. Wing, and R.T. Hyde. "Chronic Disease in Former College Students XIII. Early Precursors of Peptic Ulcer." *American Journal of Epidemiology* 100:307, 1974.

Palmer, E.D. "Brief Review. Hereditary Aspects of Ulcer Disease." *Gastrointestinal Endoscopy* 16:163, 1970.

Palmer, W.L. "Peptic Ulcer." In M. Paulson, ed., *Gastroenterologic Medicine*. Philadelphia: Lea & Febiger, 1969.

SOURCES AND SUPPLEMENTARY READING

Pereira-Lima, J., and F. Hollander. "Gastric Acid Rebound. A Review." *Gastroenterology* 37:145, 1959.

Pflanz, M. "Epidemiological and Sociocultural Factors in the Etiology of Duodenal Ulcer." *Advances in Psychosomatic Medicine* 6:121, 1971.

————, E. Rosenstein and Th. von Uexküll. "Socio-psychological Aspects of Peptic Ulcer." *Journal of Psychosomatic Research* 1:68, 1956.

————, and Th. von Uexküll. "Entlastung als pathogenetischer Faktor." *Klinische Wochenschrift* 414, 1952.

Pilot, M.L., A. Muggia, and H.M. Spiro. "Duodenal Ulcer in Women." *Psychosomatic Medicine* 29:586, 1967.

Piper, D.W. "Milk in the Treatment of Gastric Disease." *American Journal of Clinical Nutrition* 22:191, 1969.

Porter, R.W., J.V. Brady, D. Conrad et al. "Some Experimental Observations on Gastrointestinal Lesions in Behaviorally Conditioned Monkeys." *Psychosomatic Medicine* 20:379, 1958.

Pulvertaft, C.N. "Peptic Ulcer in Town and Country." *British Journal of Preventive and Social Medicine* 13:131, 1959.

Puri, P., and E. Boyd. "Children with Duodenal Ulcers and Their Families." *Archives of Disease in Childhood* 50:485, 1975.

Ravitch, M.M. "Duodenal Ulcer in Childhood." *Medical Times* 97(7):196, 1969.

————, and G.D. Duremdes. "Operative Treatment in Duodenal Ulcer in Childhood." *Annals of Surgery* 171:641, 1970.

————, and ————. "Operative Treatment of Duodenal Ulcer in Childhood." *Annals of Allergy* 34:145, 1975.

Redwitz, E., and H. Fuss. *Die Pathogenese des peptischen Geschwurs des Magens und der oberen Darm Abschnitte.* Stuttgart: Ferdinand Enke, 1928.

Robb, J.D.A., P.S. Thomas, J. Orszulock, and G.W. Odling-Smee. "Duodenal Ulcer in Children." *Archives of Disease in Childhood* 47:688, 1972.

Roberts, J.A.F. "ABO Blood Groups, Secretor Status, and Susceptibility to Chronic Diseases." In J.V. Neel, M.W. Shaw, and W.J. Schull, eds., *Genetics and the Epidemiology of Chronic Diseases.* U.S. Public Health Service Publication

No. 1163. Washington, D.C.: U.S. Government Printing Office, 1965.

Robinson, S.C., and M. Brucer. "The Body Build of the Male Ulcer Patient." *American Journal of Digestive Diseases* 7: 365, 1940.

Rogers, F.A. "Factors Affecting the Mortality from Gastroduodenal Perforation." *Surgery, Gynecology and Obstetrics* 111: 771, 1960.

————, and N. Hiatt. "The Natural History of Perforated Peptic Ulcer." *Medical Times* 87:367, 1959.

Rosenlund, M.L., and C.E. Koop. "Diagnosis and Treatment: Duodenal Ulcer in Childhood." *Pediatrics* 45:283, 1970.

Roth, H.P. "The Peptic Ulcer Psychology." *Archives of Internal Medicine* 96:32, 1955.

————, and H.S. Caron. "Patients' Misconceptions About Their Peptic Ulcer Diets: Potential Obstacles to Cooperation." *Journal of Chronic Diseases* 20:5, 1967.

Roth, J.L.A. "Clinical Evaluation of the Caffeine Gastric Analysis in Duodenal Ulcer Patients." *Gastroenterology* 19:199, 1951.

————. "Symptomatology (Ulcer)." In H.L. Bockus, ed., *Gastroenterology,* 2nd ed. Philadelphia: W.B. Saunders, 1963.

————. "The Ulcer Patient Should Watch His Diet." In F.J. Ingelfinger et al., eds., *Controversy in Internal Medicine.* Philadelphia: W.B. Saunders, 1966.

Saint-Hilaire, S.M., M. Lavers, J. Kennedy, and C. Code. "Gastric Acid Secretory Value of Different Foods." *Gastroenterology* 39:1, 1960.

Sandweiss, D.J., H.C. Saltzstein, and A.A. Forbman. "The Relation of Sex Hormones to Peptic Ulcer." *American Journal of Digestive Diseases* 6:6, 1939.

Schanke, K. "The Behavior of Gastric and Duodenal Ulcer in a Fishing District in the North of Norway." *Acta Chirurgica Scandinavica,* Supplement 115, 1946.

Scott, H.W., Jr., J.L. Sawyers, W.G. Gobbel, Jr., et al. "Definitive Surgical Treatment in Duodenal Ulcer Disease. E. Duodenal Ulcer in Infants and Children." *Current Problems in Surgery,* October 1968, pp. 38–39.

Segi, M., S. Fujisaku, and M. Kurichara. "Mortality of Duodenal and Gastric Ulcer in Countries and Its Geographical Correlation to Mortality of Gastric and Intestinal Cancer." *Schweiserische Leitschrift Fur Allgemeine Pathologie* 22: 777, 1959.

Selye, H. *Stress: The Physiology and Pathology of Exposure to Stress.* Montreal: Acta, 1950.

Shaper, A.G., and A.W. Williams. "Peptic Ulcer in Africans." *British Medical Journal* 2:757, 1959.

Shay, H., and D.C.H. Sun. "Etiology and Pathology of Gastric and Duodenal Ulcer." In H.L. Bockus, ed., *Gastroenterology,* 2nd ed. Philadelphia: W.B. Saunders, 1963.

————, and ————. "Management of Uncomplicated Peptic Ulcer." In H.L. Bockus, ed., *Gastroenterology,* 2nd ed. Philadelphia: W.B. Saunders, 1963.

Shore, J.H., and D.L. Stone. "Duodenal Ulcer Among Northwest Coastal Indian Women." *American Journal of Psychiatry* 130:774, 1973.

Sievers, M.L., and J.R. Marquis. "Duodenal Ulcer Among Southwestern American Indians." *Gastroenterology* 42:567, 1962.

Silverman, A.J., S.I. Cohen, F. Magnusson, and E. McGough. "Psychologic Factors in Gynecologic Surgery." *North Carolina Medical Journal* 17:69, 1956.

Sippy, B.W. In J.H. Musser and A.O.J. Kelly, eds., *A Handbook of Practical Treatment,* Vol. 3. Philadelphia: W.B. Saunders, 1912.

Smith, L.A. "Interpretation of Abdominal Pain." In M. Paulson, ed., *Gastroenterologic Medicine.* Philadelphia: Lea & Febiger, 1969.

Spicer, C.C., D.N. Stewart, and D.M. de R. Winser. "Perforated Peptic Ulcer During the Period of Heavy Air-raids." *Lancet* 1:19, 1944.

Spiro, H.M. *Clinical Gastroenterology.* New York and London: Macmillan, 1970.

————, R.D. Schwartz, and M.L. Pilot. "Peptic Ulcer in Pregnancy. A Serial Study of Gastric Secretion During Pregnancy." *American Journal of Digestive Diseases* 4:289, 1959.

Stein, A., M.R. Kaufman, H.D. Janowitz et al. "Changes in

SOURCES AND SUPPLEMENTARY READING

Hydrochloric Acid Secretion in a Patient with a Gastric Fistula During Intensive Psychotherapy." *Psychosomatic Medicine* 24:427, 1962.

Stewart, D.N., and D.M. de R. Winser. "Incidence of Perforated Peptic Ulcer: Effect of Heavy Air-raids." *Lancet* 1:259, 1942.

Sultz, H.A., E.R. Schlesinger, J.G. Feldman, and W.E. Mosher. "The Epidemiology of Peptic Ulcer in Childhood." *American Journal of Public Health* 60:492, 1970.

Sun, D.C.H. "Long-term Anticholinergic Therapy for Prevention of Recurrence in Duodenal Ulcer." *American Journal of Digestive Diseases* 9:706, 1964.

————. "Tests Employed in the Study of Gastric Function and Disease." In H.L. Bockus, ed., *Gastroenterology,* 2nd ed. Philadelphia: W.B. Saunders, 1963.

Susser, M. "Causes of Peptic Ulcer: A Selective Epidemiologic Review." *Journal of Chronic Diseases* 20:435, 1967.

Szasz, T.S., et al. "The Role of Hostility in the Pathogenesis of Peptic Ulcer. Theoretical Considerations with Report of a Case." *Psychosomatic Medicine* 9:331, 1947.

Thoroughman, J.C., G.R. Pascal, J.R. Jarvis, and J.C. Crutcher. "A Study of Psychological Factors in Patients with Surgically Intractable Duodenal Ulcer and Those with Other Intractable Disorders." *Psychosomatic Medicine* 29:233, 1967.

Tovey, F.I. "Geographic Distribution of Peptic Ulcers." *Tropical Doctor* 4:17, 1974.

————. "An Investigation of the Buffering Action and the Effect on Pepsin of Bran and Unrefined Carbohydrate Foods." *Postgraduate Medical Journal* 50:683, 1974.

————, A.P. Jayaraj, and C.G. Clark. "The Possibility of Dietary Protective Factors in Duodenal Ulcer." *Postgraduate Medical Journal* 51:366, 1975.

————, and M. Tunstall. "Duodenal Ulcer in Black Populations in Africa South of the Sahara." *Gut* 16:564, 1975.

Tudor, R.B. "Peptic Ulcerations in Childhood." *Pediatric Clinics of North America* 14:109, 1967.

Ukers, W.H. *All About Coffee.* New York: Tea and Coffee Trade Journal Co., 1935.

SOURCES AND SUPPLEMENTARY READING

Viskum, K. "Mind and Ulcer." *Acta Psychiatrica Scandinavica* 51:182, 1975.

Walsh, J.H. "Control of Gastric Secretion." In M.H. Sleisenger and J.S. Fordtran, eds., *Gastrointestinal Disease.* Philadelphia: W.B. Saunders, 1973.

Webster, C.U., and R.D. Weir. "Perforated Peptic Ulcer in North-east Scotland." *Scottish Medical Journal* 3:288, 1958.

Weiner, H., M. Thaler, M.F. Reiser, and I.A. Mirsky. "Etiology of Duodenal Ulcer. I. Relation of Specific Psychological Characteristics to Rate of Gastric Secretion. (Serum Pepsinogen)." *Psychosomatic Medicine* 19:1, 1957.

Weir, R.D. "Perforated Peptic Ulcer in North-east Scotland." *Scottish Medical Journal* 5:257, 1960.

Welsh, J.D., and S. Wolf. "Geographical and Environmental Aspects of Peptic Ulcer." *American Journal of Medicine* 29: 754, 1960.

Williams, C.B., A.P. Forrest, and H. Campbell. "Buffering Capacity of Food in Relation to Stimulation of Gastric Secretion." *Gastroenterology* 55:567, 1968.

Wolf, S., and H.G. Wolff. *Human Gastric Function.* New York: Oxford University Press, 1947.

——, and ——. "Life Situations, Emotions, and Gastric Function. A Summary . . ." *Translations and Studies of the College of Physicians of Philadelphia* 16:97, 1948.

Wolowitz, H.M. "Oral Involvement in Peptic Ulcer." *Journal of Consulting Psychology* 31:418, 1967.

——, and S. Wagonfeld. "Oral Derivatives in the Food Preferences of Ulcer Patients. An Experimental Test of Alexander's Hypothesis." *Journal of Nervous and Mental Diseases* 146:18, 1968.

Woodward, E.R. *The Postgastrectomy Syndrome.* Springfield, Ill.: Charles C Thomas, 1963.

—— et al. "Alcohol as a Gastric Secretory Stimulant." *Gastroenterology* 32:727, 1957.

Work Group XI. "Psychosocial Forces." *Gastroenterology* 69: 1161, 1975.

Wretmark, G. "Mental and Psychosomatic Morbidity in Peptic Ulcer Families." *Journal of Psychosomatic Research* 5:21, 1960.

229

SOURCES AND SUPPLEMENTARY READING

———. "The Peptic Ulcer Individual. A Study in Heredity, Physique, and Personality." *Acta Psychiatrica et Neurologica Scandinavica* Supplement 84, 1953, pp. 1–183.

Yager, J., and H. Weiner. "Peptic Ulcer. Observations in Man with Remarks on Pathogenesis." *Advances in Psychosomatic Medicine* 6:40, 1971.

Index

M. MICHAEL EISENBERG was born in New York City in 1931. He received his M.D. degree with honors from the Harvard Medical School in 1956 and took his surgical training at the Peter Bent Brigham Hospital in Boston and at the Yale New Haven Medical Center. He received additional clinical and research training in gastrointestinal diseases at the University of Florida and the University of California in Los Angeles and was made associate professor of surgery at the University of Florida in 1967. He became professor and head of gastrointestinal surgery at the University of Minnesota in 1968, where he still teaches and practices.

He has lectured in universities from California to Moscow and has published over a hundred articles and books on ulcers and stomach physiology.

He was recently elected president of the American Section of the International College of Surgery of the Digestive Tract. He resides in Minneapolis with his wife and three daughters.